NUTRITION AND DIET RESEARCH PROGRESS SERIES

NUTRITIONAL EDUCATION

NUTRITION AND DIET RESEARCH PROGRESS SERIES

Diet Quality of Americans
Nancy Cole and Mary Kay Fox
2009. ISBN: 978-1-60692-777-9

Diet Quality of Americans
Nancy Cole and Mary Kay Fox
2009. ISBN: 978-1-60876-499-0 (Online Book)

School Nutrition and Children
Thomas J. Baxter (Editor)
2009. ISBN: 978-1-60692-891-2

Appetite and Nutritional Assessment
Shane J. Ellsworth and Reece C. Schuster (Editors)
2009. ISBN: 978-1-60741-085-0

Beta Carotene: Dietary Sources, Cancer and Cognition
Leiv Haugen and Terje Bjornson (Editors)
2009. ISBN: 978-1-60741-611-1

Flavonoids: Biosynthesis, Biological Effects and Dietary Sources
Raymond B. Keller (Editor)
2009. ISBN: 978-1-60741-622-7

Handbook of Vitamin C Research: Daily Requirements, Dietary Sources and Adverse Effects
Hubert Kucharski and Julek Zajac (Editors)
2009. ISBN: 978-1-60741-874-0

Supercritical Fluid Technology Applied to the Manufacture of Prebiotic Carbohydrates
Tiziana Fornari, Fernando Montañés, Agustín Olano and Elena Ibáñez
2010. ISBN: 978-1-60876-978-0

Biological Effects of β -Carotene
Rosa Martha Perez Gutierrez, Adriana Maria Neira Gonzalez and Sandra Lugardo Diaz
2010. ISBN: 978-1-61668-256-9

Biological Effects of β -Carotene
Rosa Martha Perez Gutierrez, Adriana Maria Neira Gonzalez and Sandra Lugardo Diaz
2010. ISBN: 978-1-61668-609-3 (Online book)

Nutritional Education
Ida R. Laidyth (Editor)
2010. ISBN: 978-1-60876-078-7

Dietary Supplements: Primer and FDA Oversight
Timothy H. Riley (Editor)
2010. ISBN: 978-1-60741-891-7

Handbook of Nutritional Biochemistry: Genomics, Metabolomics and Food Supply
Sondre Haugen and Simen Meijer (Editors)
2010. ISBN: 978-1-60741-916-7

Dietary Fiber, Fruit and Vegetable Consumption and Health
Friedrich Klein and Georg Möller (Editors)
2010. ISBN: 978-1-60876-025-1

Maintaining a Healthy Diet
Anna R. Bernstein (Editor)
2010. ISBN: 978-1-60741-856-6

Nutritional Factors and Osteoporosis Prevention
Masayoshi Yamaguchi
2010. ISBN: 978-1-60876-929-2

Vitamin D: Biochemistry, Nutrition and Roles
William J. Stackhouse (Editor)
2010. ISBN: 978-1-61668-273-6

Vitamin D: Biochemistry, Nutrition and Roles
William J. Stackhouse (Editor)
2010. ISBN: 978-1-61668-713-7 (Online book)

Phytochemicals for the Control of Human Appetite and Body Weight
S.A. Tucci, E.J. Boyland and J.C. Halford
2010. ISBN: 978-1-61668-676-5

Phytochemicals for the Control of Human Appetite and Body Weight
S.A. Tucci, E.J. Boyland and J.C. Halford
2010. ISBN: 978-1-61668-897-4 (Online book)

NUTRITION AND DIET RESEARCH PROGRESS SERIES

NUTRITIONAL EDUCATION

IDA R. LAIDYTH
EDITOR

Nova Science Publishers, Inc.
New York

For permission to use material from this book please contact us:
Telephone 631-231-7269; Fax 631-231-8175
Web Site: http://www.novapublishers.com

LIBRARY OF CONGRESS CATALOGING-IN-PUBLICATION DATA
Nutritional education / [edited by] Ida R. Laidyth.
p. cm.
ISBN 978-1-60876-078-7 (hardcover)
1. Nutrition--Study and teaching. 2. Obesity--Prevention--Study and teaching. 3. Health promotion. I. Laidyth, Ida R.
RA784.N885 2009
613.2071--dc22

2009031037

Published by Nova Science Publishers, Inc. ✢ New York

CONTENTS

PREFACE

Nutritional education programs have been implemented in the workplace and in schools in an effort to improve diet and lifestyle, and therefore, reduce the incidence of many chronic diseases linked to overweight and obesity including; diabetes, cardiovascular disease and cancer. Providing age-appropriate, culturally sensitive instruction and materials were connected to the success of nutritional education programs. This new and important book gathers the latest research from around the globe in the study of nutritional education and highlights such topics as: nutrition education in the workplace, metabolic syndrome in children, school feeding programs, maternal nutritional education during pregnancy, nutrition and tuberculosis, nutrition education in school-based childhood and adolescent programs, and others.

Chapter 1 - Reviews of the existing evidence have demonstrated the effectiveness of lifestyle interventions in producing a modest total weight loss amongst overweight and obese adults. However, there is a dearth of research to explore the experiences of these individuals, or to obtain their views on the feasibility and acceptability of the educational messages delivered. This chapter seeks to add to the qualitative evidence base regarding the perceptions of adults who receive nutritional education as part of treatment for overweight and obesity. The authors have drawn together the findings from two qualitative studies conducted in the North East of England to explore the lived experience of individuals participating in non-commercial weight loss programmes. The programmes in question were delivered in primary care or community settings and targeted adults from socio-economically disadvantaged backgrounds. A number of barriers and facilitators to implementing the lessons learned have been identified and considered in light of the existing theoretical and empirical literature. The chapter concludes with a discussion of the implications of these findings for policy, practice and future research.

Chapter 2- Nutrition education programs have been implemented in the workplace in an effort to improve the diet and lifestyle of employees and, therefore, reduce the incidence of many chronic diseases linked to overweight and obesity including, diabetes, cardiovascular disease and cancer. Despite the importance of this outcome, the success of these programs has varied. This chapter uses a qualitative, narrative approach to review research conducted over the past 10 years on nutrition programs in the workplace and attempts to identify those aspects associated with successful behaviour change among employees. This approach enables us to include a variety of methods of intervention and data collection and thereby allows identification of promising intervention approaches that might not be identified in review approaches that are based on quantitative meta-analyses.

The chapter reviews the evidence for both the efficacy and the effectiveness of nutrition education programs in the workplace (i.e., whether an intervention works under ideal, well controlled conditions, versus whether the intervention works in the "uncontrolled" real-world workplace) (Spraycar, 1995). In addition, the characteristics of efficacious and effective programs are described including the duration of the nutrition education programs, the type of programs offered to employees, and the settings in which the programs were implemented. The results of the review suggest the workplace is a viable context for delivery of programs designed to change food intake behaviours, and overweight and obesity prevalence, although the challenge is to achieve sustained change on these outcomes after the intervention concludes. The results of this review should be taken into account when planning future work-based education programs on nutrition.

Chapter 3- The purpose of this chapter was to review nutrition education in school-based childhood and adolescent obesity prevention programs. Problems of overweight and obesity have reached epidemic proportions in children and adolescents. With the large number of children and adolescents affected by overweight and obesity, it has been recognized as a critical public health threat, and prevention should become a priority. Schools have been considered an important venue for the delivery of health education programs since a majority of the nation's youth can be reached. Implementing a program in the school does not necessarily correspond to success, and therefore common components among successful nutrition education programs were examined. Providing age-appropriate, culturally sensitive instruction and materials were connected to the success of the programs. Success was also found when the nutrition education program was relevant to the student, and information was applicable to their everyday life. It was also critical to go beyond dissemination of knowledge and develop attitudes, skills, and behaviors to adopt, maintain, and enjoy healthy nutrition habits. Finally, recommendations were made to enhance the effectiveness of future school-based nutrition education programs.

Chapter 4- Nutrition plays both an ongoing and fluctuating environmental role influencing gene expression and observed phenotypic variation of complex traits, such as the serum lipid transport system. Individual nutritional status is influenced by a mélange of multiple cultural, biological, generational, epigenetic and genetic factors, all of which can ultimately affect the genetic profiles of a population. Despite increasing awareness of sex-specific effects, few research studies address the mechanisms by which factors of sexual dimorphism may influence the relationship between nutrients and genes in trait expression. Not all differences can be solely attributed to the direct effect of sex hormones. The effects of body composition, metabolically active adipose tissue and its active adipokines, macronutrient energy preference and metabolism are among the potential underlying factors affecting normal sex-specific expression of nutrient-by-gene interaction on complex traits. This chapter explores the mechanisms through which both direct and indirect effects of steroid hormones may influence biomarkers of lipid metabolism. Given the emphasis on dietary manipulation of serum lipids as a primary strategy in prevention of cardiovascular disease (CVD), further research addressing aspects of sexual dimorphism underlying variation of the lipid profile is imperative. We examine current literature addressing the effects of nutrition and sexual dimorphism in body composition, fat patterning and hormones, energy homeostasis and metabolism and their association with serum lipids. Studies of dietary strategies as the first line of defense against susceptibility to disease have often concentrated on male subjects, with little understanding of female variation, and therefore having inconsistent results when applied to females.

Chapter 5- The obesity epidemic in the United States and the continuing rise in the number of children and adolescents who are overweight and have type 2 diabetes mellitus[1], as well as reports by life-course epidemiologists [2] who identify that poor health in childhood can lead to acute and chronic illness in adulthood, provide evidence that the presence of metabolic syndrome in children and adolescents is a risk factor for developing cardiovascular disease and type 2 diabetes[3]. The purpose of this paper is threefold: (1) To review the risk factors for developing metabolic syndrome in children and adolescents; (2) to report on the projected long-term health effects of metabolic syndrome; and (3) to describe health and wellness programs that have been implemented to address the rise in overweight children and adolescents at risk for metabolic syndrome, cardiovascular disease, and type 2 diabetes mellitus.

Chapter 6- The paper reviews methods for enhancing learning at tertiary level by using information technology, including published examples relevant to nutrition education of adults in other contexts. Teaching may include animations that enhance understanding and personal response systems that provide immediate feedback about student comprehension. Tutorials, practical classes and self-study materials can incorporate a wide range of computer programs. These have been used for many years to permit students to analyse their own diets, which is known to provide useful feedback to enable changes to be made. Students learn from exercises in which they have to improve diets and they can become more familiar with food composition using computer-generated bar charts in a quiz format. Programs can integrate energy expenditure with different levels of activity to energy intake with different diets. Students may learn how vitamins are involved in metabolism by exploring pathways using an interactive program. Student research projects can be enhanced by using a program that helps them write a protocol and the output of statistical programs can be interpreted by a program that reads the screen and explains what it means. Computers can be used as vehicles for simulations of practical situations such as client interviews and they can provide discussion forums for students on placement. Whilst revising before assessments, students may benefit from a variety of testing programs; for example crossword puzzles test their knowledge in an enjoyable way and construction of sentences using words from a list tests their understanding of concepts.

Chapter 7- School Feeding Programs have been established in most parts of the world with the goals of reducing hunger and malnutrition. School Feeding Programmes have potential to safeguard the health and the well-being of school children, and also promote good dietary, hygiene, and sanitation practices. School children grow up knowing the consumption of nutritious commodities and other foods. School Feeding Programs have been used as a means to distribute food to the pre-school and school-age children, as a food security net to improve their nutrition status, and also improve the general socio-economic conditions of rural communities as well as providing educational and nutritional benefits of participants. Nutrition status is a powerful determinant of educational health and developmental outcomes of school children. Nutrition status affects physical growth and maturation, and influences a person's attention span, learning capacity and ability to engage in educational experience. Undernutrition in early childhood has potential to negatively influence school aptitudes, time of school enrollment, school attendance and concentration. Schools provide an ideal channel for nutrition programs and services especially now that they reach many children. Acceptable dietary, hygiene and sanitation habits can be developed amongst school children in school. Most children from resource-poor households are often absent from schools as they provide child labor on farms and households to augment their families much needed income for food purchases. The development of health-promoting schools has promising returns for school children in developing countries. This study demonstrates the interaction of poverty, nutrition status and education. To improve the nutritional status and school attendance of the pupils whose parents cannot afford to participate in the School Lunch Programs, funding from external sources is essential. Efforts should be directed toward reducing hunger in the classroom and improving the nutritional status of pupils in schools. Inclusion of School Feeding Programs as a policy issue in national goals and objectives could result in improved nutritional status among school children.

Chapter 8- Maternal nutritional status before and during pregnancy constitutes one of the most important determinants for fetal growth. In adequate body weight before conception and low maternal weight gain are associated with adverse perinatal outcomes. The fetal origins hypothesis proposes that inadequate maternal nutrition and a low infant birth weight can predispose the child to diseases such as, diabetes and cardiovascular disease later in life. Pregnancy can be an opportune time to improve nutrition, and presents an ideal time for health promotion activities. However, many women of childbearing age do not maintain good nutritional status before and during pregnancy. They do not have an opportunity to get adequate and appropriate nutrition education in antenatal care. Most of them expect advice on general dietary improvements, with the remainder seeking advice on helping to promote their quality and quantity of nutritional intake. All women of reproductive age should be encouraged to follow the Government recommendation and eat a well-balanced diet. Health care providers need to ensure pregnant women know the positive and negative effect of poor maternal nutrition status, including the need for additional folate, at each physical check-up. An individualized approach is likely to have better outcomes than a standard intervention that is given to all pregnant women. A critical goal to achieve is for women to make behavior changes for good nutritional status before, during, and beyond pregnancy, which may lead to improved birth outcomes.

Chapter 9- Evidences are accumulating in both human and animal studies that undernutrition is associated with increased risk and severity of tuberculosis. In addition, obesity appears to protect against tuberculosis. Diabetes mellitus increases risk of tuberculosis, but poor diabetic control contributes to the bulk of such risk. In both under-nutrition and poor diabetic control, the increased risk is seen mainly in the pulmonary form of the disease, and the exact reason for relative sparing of the extrapulmonary sites remains unclear. Undernutrition has also been associated with worsened prognosis, poorer response to treatment and increased risk of relapse. Data from randomized controlled trials are scanty, as nutritional supplementation trials are often costly and difficult to implement. Micronutrients have been shown to decrease the risk of reversion of sputum culture to positivity after initial conversion, but there was no significant effect on mortality. With the putative roles of systemic inflammatory responses in tuberculosis manifestations, adjunctive corticosteroid administration treatment has been found to afford earlier and more significant body weight gain, albeit no differences in sputum bacteriological conversion and disease relapse rate. Further studies, with better study designs and serial monitoring of relevant nutritional parameters, are required to clarify the complex situation.

Chapter 10- Evidences are accumulating in both human and animal studies that undernutrition is associated with increased risk and severity of tuberculosis. In addition, obesity appears to protect against tuberculosis. Diabetes mellitus increases risk of tuberculosis, but poor diabetic control contributes to the bulk of such risk. In both under-nutrition and poor diabetic control, the increased risk is seen mainly in the pulmonary form of the disease, and the exact reason for relative sparing of the extrapulmonary sites remains unclear. Undernutrition has also been associated with worsened prognosis, poorer response to treatment and increased risk of relapse. Data from randomized controlled trials are scanty, as nutritional supplementation trials are often costly and difficult to implement. Micronutrients have been shown to decrease the risk of reversion of sputum culture to positivity after initial conversion, but there was no significant effect on mortality. With the putative roles of systemic inflammatory responses in tuberculosis manifestations, adjunctive corticosteroid administration treatment has been found to afford earlier and more significant body weight gain, albeit no differences in sputum bacteriological conversion and disease relapse rate. Further studies, with better study designs and serial monitoring of relevant nutritional parameters, are required to clarify the complex situation.

In: Nutritional Education
Editor: Ida R. Laidyth

ISBN: 978-1-60876-078-7

Chapter 1

Exploring the Views and Experiences of Participants in Structured Weight Loss Programmes

***S. Visram*[1] *and A. Crosland*[2]**

[1] Postgraduate Research Associate (BA Hons, MA Oxon, MPH), Community, Health and Education Studies (CHESs) Research Centre, Northumbria University, Newcastle-upon-Tyne, England.

[2] Professor of Nursing (RGN, MA, PhD), Faculty of Applied Sciences, University of Sunderland, Sunderland, England.

Abstract

Reviews of the existing evidence have demonstrated the effectiveness of lifestyle interventions in producing a modest total weight loss amongst overweight and obese adults. However, there is a dearth of research to explore the experiences of these individuals, or to obtain their views on the feasibility and acceptability of the educational messages delivered. This chapter seeks to add to the qualitative evidence base regarding the perceptions of adults who receive nutritional education as part of treatment for overweight and obesity. The authors have drawn together the findings from two qualitative studies conducted in the North East of England to explore the lived experience of individuals participating in non-commercial weight loss programmes. The programmes in question were delivered in primary care or community settings and targeted adults from socio-economically disadvantaged backgrounds. A number of barriers and facilitators to implementing the lessons learned have been identified and considered in light of the existing theoretical and empirical literature. The chapter concludes with a discussion of the implications of these findings for policy, practice and future research.

INTRODUCTION

Obesity is widely considered to be one of the greatest global public health challenges of the 21st century, with more than one billion adults overweight and at least 300 million clinically obese (WHO, 2004). Although the mechanism of obesity development is not fully understood, it is known that the condition occurs when energy intake exceeds energy expenditure, and that environmental factors, cultural practices and lifestyle preferences all play a major role in its rising prevalence worldwide (Institute of Nutrition Metabolism and Diabetes, 2003). Obesity has overtaken smoking to become the number one public health issue in England, with 24 million adults – more than half of the country's adult population – considered to exceed the healthy weight for their height (Joint Health Surveys Unit, 2004). Since the 1980s the number of adults in England classified as clinically obese has more than doubled, with 24 per cent of men and women over 16 years of age falling into this category (The Health and Social Care Information Centre, 2009). Figure 1 provides an illustration of the most recent national statistics on adult overweight and obesity, and also demonstrates the trends over time for men and women. Levels of adult obesity across Europe and the USA are expected to increase further as a result of the rising prevalence of childhood obesity in recent decades (Troiano & Flegel, 1998). Around 80 per cent of obese children and adolescents go on to become obese adults, adding to the burden of excess weight amongst adults which has reached epidemic proportions on a global scale (Whitaker et al., 1997; WHO, 2004).

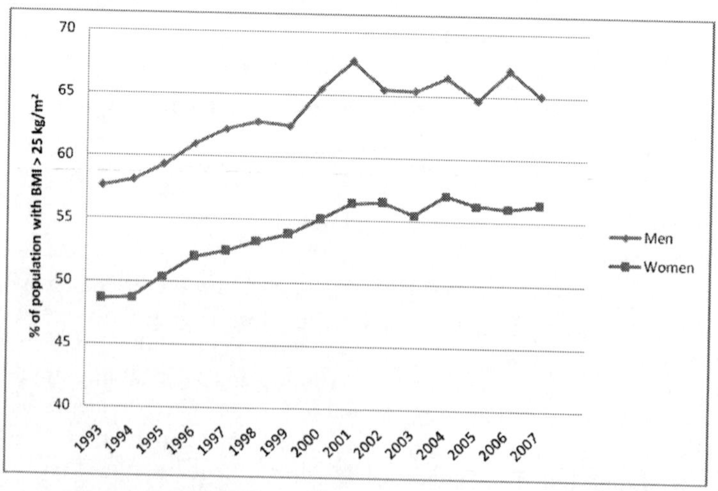

Figure 1. Trends in Adult Overweight and Obesity in England (1993 – 2007)

In the clinical environment, obesity tends to be measured using techniques such as waist circumference, skin fold thickness and body mass index (BMI), which is defined as body weight in kilograms divided by the square of height in metres (kg/m^2) (Kopelman, 2000). A person with a BMI between 25 and 30 kg/m^2 is classed as being overweight and a person with a BMI over 30 kg/m^2 is considered to be clinically obese (WHO, 2000). This measure allows meaningful comparisons of weight status within and between populations and the identification of individuals and groups at risk of morbidity and mortality. However, BMI fails to distinguish between fat and fat-free mass (muscle and bone) and therefore cannot take body shape or fat distribution into account. Epidemiological and metabolic studies have shown that the complications of obesity are more closely related to the distribution of excess fat rather than overall excess weight (Despres et al., 2001). Around a third of men and women in England have an elevated waist to hip ratio, which indicates abdominal obesity and is a major risk factor for diabetes, cardiovascular disease and mortality (Joint Health Surveys Unit, 2004). There are also significant age and ethnic group differences in the accumulation of visceral adipose tissue, as well as confounding factors relating to the risk of coronary heart disease for women as opposed to men (Lean et al., 1995; Lemieux et al., 1996a; 1996b). There is evidence to suggest that the risk of overweight and obesity increases with rising social deprivation; for example, obesity is known to be more common in adults employed in manual occupations, particularly women (Reilly, Wilson, Summerbell, & Wilson, 2002). In England, one-third of women in semi-routine and routine occupations have a BMI of more than 30 kg/m^2, compared to around one-fifth of those employed in managerial and professional roles (Joint Health Surveys Unit, 2004).

Public health concerns about obesity relate to its link to numerous chronic diseases, many of which are life limiting. An estimated 9,000 premature deaths per year in England can be attributed to obesity (6 per cent of all deaths) and the lifespan of a morbidly obese adult is up to 10 years less than that of someone of lower weight, which is comparable with the effects of smoking (National Audit Office, 2001; Prospective Studies Collaboration, 2009). Being obese doubles a person's risk of all-cause mortality, coronary heart disease, stroke and type 2 diabetes, and increases their risk of some cancers, musculoskeletal problems, and loss of function (National Audit Office, 2001; National Heart Lung and Blood Institute, 1998). Figure 2 below highlights a number of the potential immediate and intermediate consequences of excess weight in adults (adapted from DWP, 2008). In addition to the physical effects, obesity has considerable social and psychological consequences, such as anxiety, depression and mood disorders, as well as financial implications (Becker et al., 2001). It has been estimated that around £3.2 billion of direct costs to the National Health Service in England could be avoided each year if the population were at a healthy weight (Allender & Rayner, 2007). Recent estimates state that the cost of treatment for diseases brought on by obesity in adults is currently £1 billion, the cost of sickness absence or loss of production directly attributable to obesity is £1.4 billion, and the cost in terms of state benefits is between £1 billion and £6 billion (Health Select Committee, 2004). Obesity is now a major contributor to the global burden of chronic disease and disability, accounting for 2 to 8 per cent of health costs and 10 to 13 per cent of deaths across the European region (WHO, 2004).

A number of recent policy documents have reinforced the urgency attached to addressing the issue of overweight and obesity. It was one of the six overarching priorities in the UK government's public health White Paper, 'Choosing Health: making healthy choices easier', which drew together a series of other initiatives such as the National Service Frameworks on Coronary Heart Disease and Diabetes, and the National Cancer Plan (Department of Health, 2004). 'Choosing Health' highlighted the need for fundamental changes to both individual lifestyles and the environment if the current obesity trend is to be halted. This was reinforced by the Foresight project, which aimed to take a strategic view of obesity in the UK and devise a sustainable, long-term response (Butland et al., 2007). It was estimated that, by 2050, the financial impact to society attributable to obesity could become an additional £45.5 billion per year. The key message of the Foresight project was that policies aimed solely at individuals will be inadequate to reverse this trend. Instead, significant effective action to prevent obesity is required at multiple levels – individual, family, community and population. In 2006, the National Institute for Health and Clinical Excellence (NICE) published the first national guidance on the prevention, identification, assessment and management of overweight and obesity in England and Wales (NICE, 2006). The guidance supports the implementation of the 'Choosing Health' White Paper and existing National Service Frameworks, and contains evidence-based recommendations for the management and prevention of overweight and obesity in both NHS and non-NHS settings. NICE has also published guidance on behaviour change, which highlights key concepts from the psychological literature that might be used to structure and inform interventions to tackle obesity (NICE, 2007). This guidance highlights the importance of being clear about the behaviours that the intervention is intending to change, the contextual changes that need to be made, and also whether the intention is to change the behaviour of individuals, communities or the wider population.

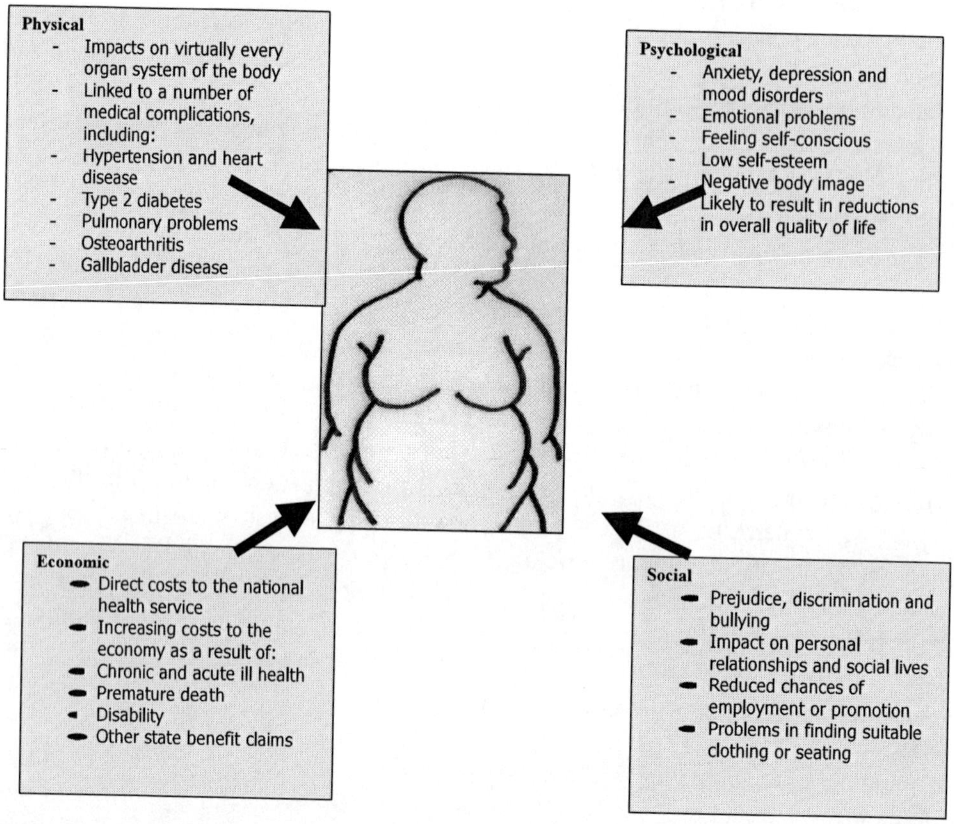

Figure 2. Consequences of Excess Weight in Adults

In spite of the policy rhetoric, most approaches to tackling obesity have focused on attempts to change the diet and exercise behaviour of individuals, rather than taking a community or population-based approach. For the treatment of obesity in adults, the aim is generally to use diet, physical activity and behavioural strategies, in combination where possible. Systematic reviews of the existing evidence have demonstrated the effectiveness of various lifestyle interventions in producing a modest total weight loss amongst adult participants (Astrup et al., 2000; Effective Health Care, 1997; Mulvihill & Quigley, 2003;

NHS Centre for Reviews and Dissemination, 1997; Pirozzo et al., 2002). However, the overall success of non-surgical approaches has been disappointing, leading some experts to conclude that treatment of obesity, which aims to establish normal bodyweight, is unrealistically optimistic (Ebbeling et al., 2002). Most interventions are marked by small changes in relative adiposity followed by substantial relapse, with some 70 per cent of successful individuals regaining at least half of the weight lost within two years (Heffernan, 2003). One explanation for this lack of success is that the dietary and physical activity prescriptions used in the majority of programmes are not particularly efficacious. Most interventions focus on reduction of fat intake, even though dietary fat might not be an important cause of obesity, and use conventional programmed exercise prescriptions, even though increasing lifestyle activity or reducing sedentary behaviours might be better for long-term weight control (Epstein et al., 1994). A second potential explanation is that adverse environmental factors overwhelm the behavioural and educational techniques designed to reduce energy intake and increase activity levels (Ebbeling et al., 2002). The term 'passive obesity' has been coined to describe the way in which the average person is likely to gain weight simply by living an ordinary life in contemporary society, as a result of the available technology, transport and food choices (Butland et al., 2007).The challenge is therefore to identify obesogenic environments and influence them so that healthier choices are more available, easier to access, and widely promoted to the whole population.

As well as gaps in the evidence base regarding the long-term effectiveness of interventions, there is a dearth of research to explore service users' views and experiences of weight management. Whilst interventions may be well intentioned, strategies for weight loss often ignore the actual causes of weight gain and the factors prompting people to attempt to control their diet. Conventional dietary studies may yield information on nutrient intake and food choice, but the benefit to public health has been limited since this knowledge is divorced from the social context of its application (Germov & Williams, 1996). Studying weight-related issues in context requires the use of qualitative research methods from a sociological perspective, an approach which has generally been neglected due to the grounding of nutrition research in the positivistic paradigm. Qualitative approaches have previously been used to explore views on becoming and being obese (Barker & Cooke, 1992; Douglas et al., 2008; Grant & Boersma, 2005; Thomas et al., 2008), experiences of stigmatisation (Cossrow et al., 2001; Rogge et al., 2004), weight loss attempts (Adolfsson et al., 2002; Bidgood & Buckroyd, 2005; Cioffi, 2002a; Jones et al., 2007), and accounts of successful weight loss and maintenance or relapse (Byrne, 2002; Byrne et al., 2003; Roberts & Ashley, 1999; Sarlio-Lahteenkorva, 1998, 2000). However, these studies remain relatively rare considering the growing interest in obesity and the increasing recognition that lay people are 'experts' in their own lives (Popay & Williams, 1996; Sarlio-Lahteenkorva, 2000). Overweight and obese people are likely to have valuable insights into weight-related issues, which may be used to enhance the effectiveness, acceptability and equity of service provision. The research described in this chapter is an attempt to increase our knowledge about people's lived experiences of obesity treatment and how the lessons learned impact upon their lives.

RESEARCH SETTING

We have sought to add to the existing evidence base around views of nutritional education by comparing and contrasting data from two qualitative studies conducted in the North East of England. The health of people in the North East is generally worse than for England as a whole and, compared with other regions, it has the highest levels of deprivation, lowest life expectancy and highest rate of early deaths from cancer (APHO, 2008a). In terms of lifestyles, the region has the highest estimated levels of adult binge drinking and smoking, and lowest levels of healthy eating and physical activity in the country. Regional data from 2003 showed that the prevalence of obesity amongst men was 23.0% (1.3% of whom were morbidly obese) and for women was 24.3% (1.6% morbidly obese) (NEPHO, 2007). By 2008, the overall prevalence of adult obesity in the North East had risen to 25.2% compared with the national average of 23.6%, representing the third highest prevalence in England (APHO, 2008a). The principal city in the region is Newcastle-upon-Tyne, which is marked by wide socioeconomic contrasts. Men from the least deprived areas of the city can expect to live approximately nine years longer than those from the most deprived areas, whereas women can expect to live about six years longer (APHO, 2008b). Although Newcastle has a lower than average prevalence of adult obesity (22.6%), the estimated level of healthy eating is significantly poorer than for England as a whole (20.3% of the local population, compared with 26.3% nationally). Over the last ten years, death rates from all causes have decreased for men and women in Newcastle, yet all rates remain above the national averages (APHO, 2008a).

The local primary health care trust in Newcastle developed the Specialist Weight Management Service (SWiMS) to provide structured support and nutritional education to adults with a BMI above 25kg/m^2, with one or more existing co-morbidities, and living in areas of socio-economic deprivation across the city. The service complemented existing Level 1 provision (targeting the general population) offered by Newcastle Primary Care Trust, by providing intervention at two additional levels: Level 2 (targeting overweight and obese individuals with existing co-morbidities) and Level 3 (targeting morbidly obese individuals, i.e. those with a BMI above 40kg/m^2). The Level 2 intervention comprised eight consecutive weekly meetings and four follow-up meetings at monthly intervals, with input from a nurse specialist, dietician or nutrition worker, exercise instructor and, where necessary, a psychologist. Participants were seen at a primary health care clinic and other local venues in groups of between 15 and 20 people, then supported at a distance by the service at three months and at six months. Level 3 participants were offered the option of either attending the group sessions or being seen on a one-to-one basis by the nurse specialist either at home or in the clinic. Individuals seen at home usually had a co-existing serious health or social problem which meant they were unwilling or unable to attend the clinic, and therefore received an intervention tailored to their needs. SWiMS also had links with tertiary care services and could refer directly for assessment of the need for gastric surgery, as well as being able to supply anti-obesity medication. The service began as a pilot in November 2002 and was designed in light of the best available evidence regarding the treatment of overweight and obesity in adults, and management of their co-morbidities (Wanless, 2004).

In contrast, the 'Balance it! It's Your Health' programme[1] in Gateshead was informed by a social marketing approach and developed in response to locally conducted research, which identified the need for a holistic and accessible service to help overweight and obese people to lose weight (SMS, 2004, 2006). The programme, which began as a pilot in April 2007, was delivered in partnership between the local health care trusts, local government and community learning service. The borough of Gateshead lies on the southern bank of the River Tyne, located directly opposite the city of Newcastle and comprising a mix of rural and urban areas. The local prevalence of adult obesity (26.0%) is higher than the national average but health inequalities are less marked than those in Newcastle (APHO, 2008c). However, a number of neighbourhoods in Gateshead are characterised by significant socioeconomic deprivation and low life expectancy, particularly in the central and eastern areas of the borough. The Balance It programme was developed in an attempt to reduce levels of adult overweight and obesity specifically within these neighbourhoods. It involved a 13-week structured intervention delivered at local venues in the community, plus a further 13 weeks of support for participants. Each two-hour session of the structured intervention comprised one-to-one weighing and support from a dietician or community nutrition assistant, nutritional advice and education, cooking skills training, and exercise sessions with a physical activity development worker. The follow-up intervention was kept flexible to suit the needs of specific cohorts of participants and was delivered by community health workers. Clients were pre-assessed to ascertain eligibility using the following criteria: over 18 years of age, having a BMI of more than 25 kg/m^2 and living in specified neighbourhoods within the borough. Individuals who failed to meet one of these criteria were regularly accepted onto the programme but their results could not be used towards the target of reducing adult BMI in a particular local area of deprivation. Unlike SWiMS, having an existing co-morbidity was not one of the eligibility criteria for the Balance It programme nor did it involve the option of attending one-to-one appointments with a clinician. See Box 1 for an overview of the two interventions. The approach of the Balance It programme was grounded in the principles of community development and focused on secondary prevention of overweight and obesity, as well as primary prevention of co-morbidities. Otherwise, the two services, target populations and geographical areas were broadly similar, providing an excellent basis for comparative analysis.

Aims and Methods

The purpose of this chapter is to investigate the lived experience of individuals participating in non-commercial weight loss programmes involving nutritional education, and identify perceived barriers and facilitators to implementing the lessons learned. Qualitative approaches were utilised in order to allow the participants to describe their experiences in their own words, and interviews provided a useful way to pursue in-depth information in order to get the story behind participants' experiences (Robson, 2002). Clients from the SWiMS programme were recruited using a purposive sampling strategy in an effort to ensure diversity according to BMI, gender and area of residence within Newcastle-upon-Tyne. This

[1] From this point onwards, the 'Balance it! It's Your Health' programme is referred to as 'Balance It'. The Specialist Weight Management Service is referred to using the abbreviation 'SWiMS'.

is a specific type of non-probability sampling which maximises the researcher's ability to devise theory that takes adequate account of local conditions and values (Lincoln & Guba, 1985). Those who consented to participate in the study were invited to take part in a one-to-one interview on completion of the structured component of the intervention, i.e. after attending SWiMS for a minimum of eight weeks. A semi-structured approach was used to provide focus to the interviews but still allow the researcher to talk around the topic, thus exploring more dimensions of the phenomenon being studied than would otherwise be possible (Fielding, 1994). The study was conducted to examine motivational factors associated with weight loss and to explore participants' perceptions and experiences of SWiMS, as part of a wider service evaluation (see Cording, Visram, & Crosland, 2005, for details). A total of 20 individual or paired interviews (where both partners had taken part in the SWiMS programme) were conducted with clients who consented to take part in the study.

Box 1. An Overview of the Weight Loss Programmes

The Specialist Weight Management Service (SWiMS)

- Targeted overweight and obese adults with co-existing health and/or social problems and living in deprived communities across the city of Newcastle-upon-Tyne.
- Involved a 12-week group intervention for Level 2 participants (those with a BMI above 25kg/m^2), delivered at a primary care clinic and in local leisure facilities.
- One-to-one sessions were provided to Level 3 participants (with a BMI above 40kg/m^2) by the nurse specialist, either at the clinic or in participants' own homes.
- Anti-obesity medication and referral for gastric surgery were also offered, where necessary.
- Based on best available research evidence and cited as an example of 'good practice' of local public health work in the Wanless Report (2004, p.61).

The 'Balance It! It's Your Health' Programme

- Targeted overweight and obese adults without serious co-morbidities and living in specific neighbourhoods in the central and eastern areas of the borough of Gateshead.
- Individuals who did not meet all of the eligibility criteria could access the programme with friends or relatives, but were not counted towards the funding target.
- Involved a 13-week structured intervention, plus a further 13-weeks of support for all participants.
- Delivered in local venues identified by the target communities as being appropriate, accessible and having the necessary kitchen facilities to host the cooking skills sessions.
- Based on locally-conducted social marketing research and involved ongoing monitoring and evaluation to ensure the intervention remained tailored to the needs of participants.

Clients of the Balance It programme were recruited to a separate study using a convenience sampling approach, which is commonly used to assist in service development on the condition that the obtained results shall be 'tested' in a larger sample from the target population (Robson 2002). This involved inviting all clients in the initial programme cycle to take part in a qualitative study, which constituted part of a formative service evaluation (see Visram & Geddes, 2007, for information). The aim was to explore the ongoing support required by clients and also to gather their perceptions of accessing and participating in the programme, in order to inform future cycles of the Balance It intervention. As the programme consisted of closed groups of clients who had been meeting together for several weeks, focus group interviews were felt to be the most appropriate method to achieve the study aims. A key characteristic of this method is the insight and data produced by the interaction between individuals that enables participants to ask questions of each other, as well as to re-evaluate and reconsider their own understandings of their specific experiences (Morgan, 1997). The focus group also generates a framework of interpretation from participants' perspectives, thus avoiding inappropriate assumptions or generalisations (Kreuger, 1988). Clients were given the option of requesting an individual interview if preferred not to take part in a group discussion, but this option was not taken up by any of the participants. One focus group was conducted at each of the two local community centres used as a venue for delivering the Balance It programme, involving a total of 18 clients (n_1= 8 and n_2= 10). The main characteristics of both study samples are summarised in Table 1.

Table 1. Main Features of Participants in the Study Samples

Characteristic	SWiMS clients (n=20)	Balance It clients (n=18)
Sex Female Male	 15 (85%) 5 (15%)	 17 (94%) 1 (6%)
Age Mean Range	 46 years 21 – 70 years	 42 years 24 – 68 years
BMI category Healthy weight (18.5-25 kg/m^2) Overweight or obese (25-40 kg/m^2) Morbidly obese (>40 kg/m^2)	 0 16 (80%) 4 (20%)	 1 (6%) 13 (72%) 4 (22%)

Both studies were granted a favourable opinion from the relevant research ethics and governance committees. All participants were informed that they were free to withdraw at any point during the research and without giving a reason. The interviews and focus groups were audio-recorded with participants' informed consent and transcribed verbatim, with any identifying information removed. The transcripts were then analysed independently by the research teams and the main concepts within the data were identified. Trustworthiness of data interpretation was addressed by having all members of the research team independently analyse the transcripts, i.e. triangulation of analysis (Denzin, 1978). The main concepts within the data were originally identified using a thematic content analytical approach, whereby each phrase is examined, coded according to the themes within it and considered in terms of its context in the discussion (Boyatzis, 1998). We have re-analysed both sets of data in light of the aims of this chapter, in order to draw out common and discordant themes around the topic of nutritional education for the treatment of overweight and obesity. This involved utilising the techniques of meta-ethnography, which is a theory about how to interpretively, rather than aggregatively, derive understanding from multiple qualitative studies (Noblit & Hare, 1988). The data were pooled to explore the experiences shared by participants in the two interventions and also to highlight any differences between primary care-based and community-based approaches to obesity treatment. In the following section, we present three over-arching themes arising from this process, illustrated using a number of examples from the data and discussed in light of the existing empirical and theoretical literature.

FINDINGS

Motivation for Seeking Help with Weight Loss

In an attempt to identify potential triggers to action for weight loss, participants in both studies were asked about the factors that had motivated them to seek help. A desire to improve their personal health was given as the primary reason for accessing the weight loss programmes. The SWiMS clients were more likely to have sought help in an attempt to alleviate particular conditions or aid recovery from illness, whereas the Balance It clients were more concerned with enhancing their general health and wellbeing. This was not an unexpected finding given that the SWiMS clients suffered from a number of existing co-morbidities, such as arthritis, cardiovascular disease, respiratory problems and clinical depression, which have the potential to undergo substantial improvement when obese adults lose even relatively small amounts of weight (Jung, 1997; National Heart Lung and Blood Institute, 1998). The focus on illness rather than positive health was particularly noticeable amongst older participants, who seemed more concerned with maintaining rather than improving their health status. Weight loss is still more common than weight gain in older people and is also more likely to be associated with poor outcomes, including an increased risk of mortality, even when the older person is overweight (Ensrud et al., 2005; Newman et al., 2001; Wannamethee et al., 2005). Experts have warned against the application of evidence from studies in younger adults to the management of obesity in older people, which may do more harm than good (Visvanathan & Chapman, 2005). Our research suggests that the older participants were either aware that the risks of being overweight decrease with increasing age or that they were simply less concerned about the potential risks to their health than the younger participants. The average age of clients in the SWiMS sample was slightly higher than that of the Balance It sample, reflecting the concentration of weight-related morbidity in the older age groups and the secondary/tertiary prevention approach of the SWiMS intervention.

Concerns about health often acted as a trigger to help seeking and lifestyle change amongst the SWiMS clients, as illustrated by the following quote: “I have tried all ways to lose weight but I just didn’t have an incentive. But the health kick gave me the incentive” (SWiMS client 10). Participants mentioned taking longer than expected to recover from operations or injuries, finding it difficult to move around and feeling “fed up. I felt cooped up, swollen, couldn’t get very far. And I thought if I brought my weight down a bit it might help me a bit” (SWiMS client 5). The crucial initiating factor was often an explicit warning from a health professional or the discovery of a risk factor, resulting in health-related anxiety that assisted in attaining the ‘critical anxiety threshold’ often needed to initiate change (Prochaska & DiClemente, 1986; Roberts & Ashley, 1999). We also found that negative feelings associated with non-health related events, such as job interviews and family outings, could facilitate action to lose weight due to a belief amongst participants that overweight people are treated worse in these situations than non-overweight people. A number of SWiMS clients recalled experiences of feeling stigmatised, bullied or discriminated against by family members, health professionals and others in their social environment. For example, one participant said “my husband always put me down about my weight, called me names. I mean, he thinks he’s being horrible to be kind but he’s not” (SWiMS client 6). Previous research demonstrates that there is a widespread, culturally acceptable stereotype and negative attitude of obese people, which may impact on their personal relationships, employment prospects, healthcare provision and quality of life (Bidgood & Buckroyd, 2005; Cossrow et al., 2001; Rogge et al., 2004). The apparent tension between the detrimental effects of stigmatisation and its potentially beneficial role as a trigger to help seeking is discussed further in a separate paper (see Visram, Crosland, & Cording, in press).

It has been suggested that the most frequent factor motivating behaviour change tends to be a negative feeling, whereas weight loss is sustained largely by positive feelings about self (Roberts & Ashley, 1999). This was certainly true of the SWiMS clients but less so of participants in the Balance It study, who reported no incidences of past stigmatisation and placed greater emphasis on achieving positive health, wellbeing and fitness. A minority of Balance It clients had sought to lose weight for medical reasons, for example in preparation for a surgical procedure, but most had attended "for health reasons and for looking better. *And feeling better as well*" (Balance It clients 1 & 5). In accordance with findings from the existing literature, women in both studies were more likely than men to cite cosmetic factors as key motivators for weight loss and to report social pressures to be slim (Barker & Cooke, 1992; Cossrow et al., 2001). Female participants spoke about wanting to wear nicer clothes, shop in a wider range of clothing stores and generally feel more confident about their appearance. One participant expressed this by saying "getting ready to go anywhere is just a nightmare because I know I haven't got anything to wear, do you know what I mean? And that is a big thing as well. It doesn't matter for a man so much I don't think, but for a woman it's, you know… I've always had a choice of what I could wear. I haven't at the minute" (SWiMS client 17). The range of acceptable weight for women is known to be narrower than the acceptable weight range for men, and, whilst more men are medically defined as overweight, more women diet due to dissatisfaction with their body shape and size (Cossrow et al., 2001; Germov & Williams, 1996). This is reflected in the significantly higher proportions of women than men in both the SWiMS and Balance It programmes. Women are also more likely to be responsible for the purchase, cooking and consumption of food in the home, and therefore to take these factors into consideration when making a decision about their own dietary needs. The Balance It clients mentioned wanting to improve their cooking skills and understanding of nutrition, with some being motivated by a desire to make a positive impact on the health of their children or grandchildren. This was not given as a key motivating factor by the SWiMS clients, who instead spoke about improvements in their family's quality of life as secondary outcomes of their own enhanced fitness and mobility levels.

Recruitment to the Balance It programme took place largely via word of mouth, involving staff working with existing groups in Gateshead and promotional literature distributed in local venues. This type of community outreach approach is commonly used with marginalised or socially isolated groups who may be less likely to access primary health care and other mainstream services. The target population for Balance It, i.e. overweight and obese individuals living in socio-economically deprived areas, can be considered as falling into the 'hard to reach' category. Self-referral was the main source of recruitment to the programme, thereby enhancing the likelihood of participants exhibiting the necessary 'readiness to change' (Prochaska & DiClemente, 1986). The high level of motivation amongst clients resulted in a 100 per cent retention rate for the initial cycle of the Balance It programme, in contrast with a relatively high non-completion rate for the SWiMS programme. One participant said “we started off with 18 people and I was at a meeting with them yesterday and there were only 4 yesterday. From 18 to 4. To me that’s just wasting people’s time” (SWiMS client 6). All participants interviewed in the SWiMS study had been referred to the service by their general practitioner or practice nurse, although there was some variation as to whether this was at the individual’s request or the practitioner’s recommendation. In either case, referral by a health professional seemed to legitimise their concerns and ensure greater commitment to their weight loss efforts by adding credibility to the service. The low retention rate caused some frustration amongst those who had experienced long delays in attempting to access the SWiMS programme, which highlights the importance of exploring and resolving the client’s ambivalence to change. When an individual is feeling ambivalent about behaviour change, an overtly persuasive effort from a practitioner is likely to lead to resistance and this may have contributed to the high non-completion rate of SWiMS (Rollnick, Kinnersley, & Stott, 1993). In the case of Balance It, the delay between attending the pre-assessment appointment and commencing on the programme was not viewed as problematic and instead was seen as providing clients with an opportunity to prepare for change.

The Lived Experience of Weight Loss Programmes

Most participants in the SWiMS study sample reported initial fears about entering a new situation and feeling unsure about what to expect from the programme. These same concerns were not raised during the Balance It study, where participants often attended sessions with friends or family members, or at a local venue where they were likely to see a familiar face. The importance of providing social support to clients during weight loss interventions is reinforced by findings from the research literature. For example, a study conducted in the United States found that participants recruited to a weight management programme with their friends or family members had significantly better outcomes than those who were recruited alone and given a standard behavioural treatment (Wing & Jeffery, 1999). Taking part in group sessions was generally felt to make both programmes more enjoyable and beneficial, in terms of clients being able to support and encourage one another, and also share their knowledge and ideas about weight management. One individual expressed this by saying “I think if you did it on your own, when you come to that little issue of ‘what should I do with this? How much should I… you know, I’m not sure.’ There’s somebody you can ask and you can talk to and they’ll tell you ‘well, I did this’ or ‘I did that’ and it kind of helps you” (Balance It client 10). The groups provided a much-needed opportunity for individuals to talk to people from similar backgrounds and in similar situations, thereby helping to reduce feelings of social isolation and weight stigmatisation. However, some individuals may feel uncomfortable with the idea of taking part in group sessions, either as a result of past experiences of bullying and harassment or a general expectation of negative treatment. Previous qualitative work has shown that obese people often experience low self-esteem due to a perceived failure to conform to the social norm of being thin (Barker & Cooke, 1992; Douglas et al., 2008). Participants in the SWiMS study sample were more likely to report feeling self-conscious in comparison with the Balance It participants. Having the option to attend one-to-one sessions with a clinician as part of the Level 3 SWiMS intervention was greatly appreciated by these clients.

Participants in both samples had previously attempted to lose weight and, while many had been successful, the effects were generally short lived. One explanation given for this was the content of traditional diet plans, which were perceived to dictate what clients should and should not eat, rather than providing them with balanced advice and information. In comparison with commercial slimming groups, the SWiMS and Balance It programmes were felt to place less emphasis on dieting and weight loss, and more on lifestyle change and education. This alternative focus was viewed positively by all participants, who perceived it to be a more acceptable and sustainable way of achieving their weight loss goals. They also felt that they were less likely to get bored and give in to the temptation to 'cheat', as had been the case with previous attempts to lose weight. This is illustrated by the following quote: "it made us realise how easy it is to change, and not hard. Because sometimes I think people go on a diet and they don't change their life. They go on a diet and they lose weight and then they get sick after a while and that's when the weight comes on. It's all about change, like walking instead of taking the car. Instead of, you know… when I get bored I eat, nibble. Even just taking [the dogs] out now, I get myself away and put my mind off food" (SWiMS client 13). It was reported to be relatively simple to incorporate the recommended lifestyle changes into their everyday lives, which clients felt made them easier to incorporate and maintain. The theoretical basis of this idea comes from Social Cognitive Theory, which states that achieving smaller goals can improve the individual's sense of self-efficacy, i.e. their perceived level of behavioural control (Bandura, 1997; 1998). Increased self-efficacy has been shown to be a strong predictor for the adoption and maintenance of the behaviours involved in successful weight loss (Bandura, 1977; Clark et al., 1996; Sallis et al., 1986). Learning how to interpret the nutritional information found on food labels and judge appropriate portion sizes seemed to be the most valuable lessons from the SWiMS programme. The Balance It clients also reported significant changes in the meals they were preparing for themselves and their families, suggesting that the messages delivered by the programme were having an impact beyond its target group. One participant said "I find I take it home to the family, so as a family we're kind of going step-by-step slowly and we're eating better than what we did" (Balance It client 17).

A key factor in the perceived success of both programmes involved the use of appropriately skilled staff to deliver easy-to-understand advice and information. Comments about members of the programme teams were wholly positive, with staff being described as friendly, approachable and encouraging. Participants felt the staff were able to successfully motivate them without making them feel pressured or judged, which was perceived to be one of the advantages of Balance It and SWiMS over commercial slimming groups. The fact that the sessions were delivered by multi-disciplinary teams also inspired confidence and feelings of trust amongst clients. Although the staff were perceived to be professional and knowledgeable in their own fields, participants also appreciated their use of non-technical language and the fact that they were willing to help with any problems or queries that clients might have. One participant said "they don't baffle you with science. That's the type of thing that would worry some people. And if you don't understand something, if you say to them 'you know, I'm not sure how that's supposed to work' they will explain it all to you" (SWiMS client 5). There was particular appreciation for the continuity in the Balance It team, which was felt to allow clients to build up a rapport and trusting relationships with programme staff. This close relationship between the staff and clients resulted in a concern from some participants about disappointing the team when they failed in their weight loss efforts, although it was acknowledged that staff remained supportive regardless of the outcome. It is known that encouragement or pressure from an 'important other', such as a friend, family member or health professional, can facilitate successful behaviour change and weight loss (Azjen, 1991; Douglas et al., 2008; Jones et al., 2007). The SWiMS clients were upset when members of staff left and were replaced with new, unfamiliar faces. This disturbed the routine of the programme and cause anxiety for participants, as illustrated by the following quote: "it's the waiting for the new guy to phone and not knowing if I'm going to like that one as much as I liked the other one… I would have liked to have finished the six weeks with the person I'd got to know and got the confidence with 'cos I don't know what this is other person if going to be like and if they're going to teach me the same way, be as enthusiastic" (SWiMS client 1).

Previous research has shown that overweight and obese clients tend to respond better to interventions that are directed towards their personal needs (Heffernan, 2003). Participants in both the group and one-to-one interventions felt they had received tailored advice on nutrition, food preparation and physical activity that took their particular circumstances into account. However, as a result of the social marketing approach and community-based nature of the intervention, the Balance It clients seemed to be more engaged and have a greater sense of ownership over the programme. The high degree of flexibility within Balance It was felt to provide an opportunity to tailor the intervention to individual needs and preferences, and the staff actively encouraged clients to have an input into the content of the sessions. Participants in both programmes appreciated the variety of topics covered and the fact that they were learning something new to take home each week. The Balance It programme also incorporated practical demonstrations and cooking skills sessions, which were rated very highly by the focus group participants. They enjoyed the 'hands on' aspect of preparing food and the opportunity to taste it afterwards, which gave them an opportunity to experience different types of food as well as different ways of preparing familiar recipes. Allowing participants to have an input into the content of these sessions meant they were able to select meals they enjoyed eating and then learn how to prepare them in healthier ways. Hence, participants did not feel they were 'missing out' in the way they might on other weight loss programmes or diets. The use of visual and participatory methods was felt to be a more effective way of educating clients about healthy eating than written or verbal messages. This is illustrated by the following quote: "It's alright saying 'there's a recipe', but when you're getting shown and that you haven't really got to put salt and you haven't got to put flour in to make it thicker, you haven't got to be putting sugar in. And when you're seeing and then tasting the results afterwards, you think 'well, that's alright that'" (Balance It client 5). In contrast, some SWiMS clients reported finding it difficult to stick to the dietary advice delivered during the programme. For example, the recommended portion sizes were not always felt to be sufficient, particularly by the male participants.

The majority of participants also reported positive experiences of taking part in the physical activity components of the programmes and saw these as an integral part of their weight loss efforts. This is an important outcome because the evidence suggests that physical activity appears to complement nutritional education by increasing dietary adherence (Rodin & Plante, 1989). The exercises were felt to be suitable for individuals of all abilities and there were also a number of positive comments about the educational aspect of these sessions. For example, participants found it valuable to learn how to breathe properly and how the various exercises were affecting their bodies, in order to avoid the risk of injury or harm. This was a particular concern for the SWiMS clients, as medically vulnerable adults are often fearful of the pain or discomfort that may occur during exercise and there tends to be a perception amongst older adults that exercise is for the young (Seefeldt et al., 2002). An individual's perception of the relative benefits and costs, as well as the resulting decisional balance (benefits minus costs), are also known to be associated with exercise adoption (Marcus et al., 1994; Marcus & Owen, 1992; Marcus et al., 1992). Participants in both studies described the physical activity sessions as enjoyable and reported finding it easier to stay focused and motivated when exercising as a group compared with exercising alone. Many of the SWiMS clients had previously led sedentary lifestyles and subsequently increased their activity levels as a result of attending the programme, which often involved simple exercises within the home or walking more around the local area. Walking was the preferred activity for the Balance It clients as it could easily be incorporated into their everyday lives. There was a general feeling of having more energy and being 'on the go more', although some participants noticed specific improvements in their mobility and fitness levels. One client said "I've got my exercise bike upstairs and use that 'cos I can only walk so far. But I'm walking further and further every time I walk. Not getting out of breath as easy now" (SWiMS client 11). As a consequence of these physical effects, many participants also reported perceived increases in their self-esteem and confidence levels. Coupled with the gradual weight loss experienced by the majority of clients on both programmes, these improvements were felt to provide an incentive for participants to continue with their weight loss efforts in the longer term.

Barriers and Facilitators to Implementing the Lessons Learned

Participants were asked to identify any potential barriers and facilitators to their ongoing weight loss efforts. As stated above, the emphasis on adopting a healthy lifestyle rather than following a restrictive diet was reported to be a key advantage of the SWiMS and Balance It programmes over commercial weight loss groups. Participants had enjoyed being taught messages about healthy eating and exercise that they felt could be incorporated into their everyday lives, such as walking instead of using their cars for short journeys, consuming more fruits and vegetables, and eating less fried food. See Box 2 for a selection of quotes to illustrate the lifestyle changes reported by participants in both studies. These strategies have been successfully employed in similar weight loss programmes, along with behavioural techniques such as completing food diaries (Jones et al., 2007; Lavery & Loewy, 1993). The recommended changes were perceived to be relatively easy to implement and maintain, particularly in terms of the new cooking skills learned by the Balance It clients. The recipes were described as being quick and convenient to prepare, as illustrated by the following quote: "But what's nice is you're not weighing it, you don't have to weigh anything so it's not a chore to do it. It's just, there's your tablespoon and there's your portion of whatever, so you can do it without the hard work of weighing and counting calories" (Balance It client 10). The emphasis placed by both programmes on personal choice and enjoying all foods in moderation was felt to make the messages more sustainable than traditional restrictive diets. This holistic approach was perceived to have been a success and many participants reported feeling healthier as a result of attending the sessions. Weight loss was often described as an added bonus to learning about nutrition, exercise and health, and subsequently making positive changes within their lives. One client expressed this by saying "I think we've all said the same thing, we all feel different. We feel better within ourselves" (Balance It client 18).

Box 2. Lifestyle Changes Reported by Study Participants

Enhanced knowledge of nutrition and modified food purchasing habits

"I'm more aware of healthy eating and everything now and… I mean, I always did cook, but I think I'm putting myself out more now." (Balance It client 5)

"I look for now what I wouldn't have before, you know, where your tins with sugar on and the fats that's in and that sort of thing, you know. Well, I wouldn't have bo thered before" (SWiMS client 12)

"… basically, what we've been doing over the last couple of months is emptying the freezer and the fridges of all the rubbishy stuff and starting to put back in, you know, by reading the labels" (SWiMS client 18)

Variation in foods prepared and consumed by the whole family

"I used to eat the occasional piece of fruit every now and then. But now we buy in bulk" (SWiMS client 8)

"I still have a little treat but I eat healthier now. Try to eat more vegetables, pasta and all that. I don't have nothing fried, it was always grilled, even before. I try and keep… I've cut my drinking down, once every week I think I go out." (SWiMS client 13)

"… when we were [children] we got a bacon sandwich or a sausage for breakfast. And my [grandchildren] come up and get a poached egg now." (Balance It client 4)

Increased levels of physical and social activity

"I feel I'm getting out, seeing different people, talking to different people. So it's having really quite an impact on my life when I think about it." (SWiMS client 5)

"I've started playing golf again, which I gave up because I couldn't get around a golf course […] And I was really worried about starting again, but I got round and I felt good about it." (Balance It client 15)

"I go to the pool for the Aquafit on a Thursday morning. I've always walked quite a bit but I think I'm walking more. I borrowed this step thing from my daughter and I do that five to ten minutes twice a day. So, yeah, I think I do quite a bit more activity which I know I could have been doing beforehand, but you just need that sort of bit of motivation to get you going." (SWiMS client 9)

It is known that increasing people's knowledge of health risks and how to deal with them are rarely sufficient to motivate them to change their health-related behaviour (Department of Health, 2004). A facilitator to successful behaviour change amongst clients in the SWiMS sample involved the tangible benefits observed in their weight-related conditions, and the Balance It clients also reported improvements in their general health and wellbeing. For example, some participants reported being able to walk further or stand for longer periods of time, having more energy and generally feeling on a 'high'. Losing weight at a steady rate therefore provided an incentive for participants to continue with their weight loss efforts outside of the sessions, as illustrated by the following quote: "with the other diets that I've done before, you get so far down the line and you give up. Because [now] I can still say I'm losing weight, it's an incentive to continue to be careful" (SWiMS client 2). However, there was some disappointment with the gradual nature of the weight loss, particularly amongst participants who reported making significant lifestyle changes. Participants in the SWiMS sample took part in a six-month follow-up study which is described in greater detail elsewhere (see Cording et al., 2005), but many described themselves as being at a 'standstill' in terms of their weight loss efforts. This was generally attributed either to health problems or extraneous factors such as the weather, and could constitute a psychological barrier to their ongoing efforts to lead a healthy lifestyle. One client said "I felt unhappy with myself, put it that way… that I had been doing so well and suddenly I found it… when I thought about the way I was eating and that again and, with everything that was going on, I sort of felt a bit down about it" (SWiMS client 5). None of the participants had been regularly weighing themselves since completing the programme, which made it difficult to judge exactly how much they had achieved in terms of weight loss. Effective behaviour change is known to occur when people are able to set achievable goals, develop a method of reliably monitoring progress towards their goals and act on the basis of this feedback (Carver & Scheier, 1998). Hence, the process of being weighed each week during the interventions and recording any progress made was felt to have been a motivating factor for clients to continue in their weight loss efforts.

The main barrier to implementing the lessons learned over the longer term was felt to be the short-term nature of both interventions, which was most strongly expressed by clients in the SWiMS study sample. Many felt they needed the motivation of the group and programme staff to continue with their attempts to lose weight. Some of the SWiMS participants had kept in touch with each other at the six-month follow-up study and valued this peer support, but felt professional input was also needed. The desire for ongoing support and supervision amongst individuals attempting to lose weight has been highlighted in numerous studies (Adolfsson et al., 2002; Bidgood & Buckroyd, 2005; Cioffi, 2002b; Jones et al., 2007; Parham, 1993; Sarlio-Lahteenkorva, 1998). However, other research has suggested that there are certain characteristics which distinguish those who successfully maintain the weight lost from those who regain it, independent of the level of support provided. For example, a tendency to evaluate self-worth in terms of weight and shape, the use of eating to regulate mood and a lack of vigilance with regard to weight control are all factors associated with weight regainers as opposed to maintainers (Byrne, 2002; Kayman et al., 1990). The transformation from obese to reduced-obese is also known to be linked to personal self-image and social roles (Sarlio-Lahteenkorva, 2000). The Balance It clients were keen to meet and be weighed on a regular basis following completion of the formal programme, and expressed a need for longer term intervention. However, a number of these participants felt they could continue to meet on their own and support one another in their weight loss efforts as a result of the knowledge and confidence gained via the programme. One client said "Well, we may not need it [formal support] at the end of the 26 weeks. We should, as I say, know enough about cooking and what we've got to do and if we just support each other in this thing once a week and we do our exercises and we make our own little leaflets for us to get weighed" (Balance It client 4). Some were not confident that they could remain motivated over the longer term and concerns were also expressed about safety whilst exercising. Participants in both studies were keen to be kept aware of any new developments in nutrition and exercise, and there was a perceived need for a broker to introduce clients to new activities and environments. This was particularly the case with exercise facilities such as gyms, where there was some concern that clients might feel embarrassed and out of place.

Additional barriers identified by the participants involved local culture and cooking habits in the North East. There was a perception that the people targeted by these weight loss programmes tend to come from heavier families where being obese and overweight is the norm. When an individual loses weight, significant others may not be supportive or comfortable with this change as they may feel that questions are being raised about their own ability to successfully manage their weight. Previous research from the United States has shown that close friends and relatives often act as saboteurs to an individual's weight loss efforts, by wittingly or unwittingly creating temptations for the dieter, lowering their feelings of self-worth and intensifying their social isolation (English, 1993). It was also felt that there tends to be an emphasis in the North East on large portion sizes and 'finishing everything on the plate', which present challenges to individuals attempting to make and maintain positive lifestyle changes. One client said "It's okay being on your healthy eating in the house. It's when we leave the house and I'll go down to my sisters' and their fridges are full" (Balance It client 4). Participants were concerned more generally about the temptation offered by the wide availability of takeaway meals and junk foods in the local environment. For some individuals, and particularly working mothers, it was felt that time pressures might result in them choosing the easiest option rather than the healthiest option. The final potential barrier was cost, which was emphasised more amongst the Balance It focus group participants than by the SWiMS interviewees. The fact that both programmes were free to attend was felt to increase participants' adherence to the intervention and to the key messages delivered. An additional perceived advantage of the Balance It programme was that it involved convenient access to free childcare and exercise facilities, making it attractive to people living within the target communities. One client said "that's very important for local people because, you know, the transport needs, the childcare needs and everything else… if you can get a venue that's easy and is accessible and has childcare, you're going to win every time aren't you? Because it all helps with that comfort" (Balance It client 15). Participants had concerns about the perceived affordability of facilities and activities outside the programme and it was felt that these should be made more accessible to individuals and families on low incomes.

Conclusion

Our findings have shown that nutritional education for overweight and obese adults can be perceived in a positive light and also have a positive impact on participants' weight-related behaviours. The benefits of taking part in the non-commercial programmes were reported to include enhanced knowledge of nutrition, increased physical activity levels, consumption of a wider range of foods, and improvements in confidence and self-esteem. Participants in the SWiMS study sample were more likely to report feelings of self-consciousness, often as a result of previous experiences of weight stigmatisation. The Balance It clients reported no prior incidences of bullying or discrimination, but stated that attending sessions with friends or family members had contributed to them feeling more at ease. Health was a crucial motivating factor for participants in both studies, although there was variation as to whether their main concern was with alleviating current conditions or promoting future health. For the Balance It clients, this included a desire to improve the health of their children and grandchildren, reflecting the emphasis on family and community within the intervention. All participants in the SWiMS study sample had been referred to the programme by a health care professional, whereas many Balance It clients had self-referred or been recruited by word of mouth. Both programmes were evidence based, although Balance It was developed from locally gathered intelligence and employed a social marketing approach to ensure that the intervention was continuously tailored to meet local needs. This had helped to overcome some of the perceived barriers to weight loss, which included the cost of activities, the influence of local culture on food choices, temptation from family and friends, and time pressures. The recipe tasting sessions were rated particularly highly by the Balance It clients, as they were felt to have equipped participants with new skills and knowledge of how to prepare convenient, affordable and healthy meals. The holistic, lifestyle approach of both interventions was believed to make the messages easier to incorporate into participants' everyday lives and therefore more sustainable in the longer term. The group education and exercise sessions were found to be enjoyable, particularly in contrast with commercial slimming groups or individual diet plans. Participants valued the opportunities provided for peer support and social interaction, but felt that ongoing support and supervision from trained members of staff were critical to their ongoing weight loss efforts.

As the data presented here were originally collected for purposes other than the aims of this chapter, our analyses could be considered to represent an example of secondary research. Disadvantages to this approach include potential concerns about its accuracy and reliability, and the fact that additional information relevant to the research questions may not have been collected (Boslaugh, 2007). Although the data were collected for slightly different purposes, one of the authors (SV) was involved in both studies and therefore it has been possible to verify the credibility of the findings. Using extracts from participants' verbatim accounts also increases the dependability of the discussion by grounding our interpretations within the data. Detailed information has been provided regarding the participants, research contexts, processes of data generation and analysis, to enable readers to decide how far and to whom the findings may be transferred (Johnson, 1997). The fact that data from the two study samples were collected using different methods (i.e. individual interviews and focus groups) could also raise questions about the comparability of the findings. However, from the perspective of meta-ethnography, allowing the participants to describe their experiences, thoughts and feelings in their own words and in appropriate ways simply adds to the richness of the interpretations. The interview method enables the researcher to stay close to what happened to a person or group of people by capturing their individual and/or collective stories (Benner, 1994; Lincoln & Guba, 1985). Furthermore, the aim of meta-ethnography is to achieve greater understanding and attain a higher level of conceptual development by interpretively, rather than aggregatively, deriving understanding from multiple studies (Noblit & Hare, 1988). As the original studies were based on similar conceptual frameworks, their synthesis has been unproblematic in comparison with attempts to synthesise studies employing different perspectives and methodologies (Campbell et al., 2003). Finally, the relatively small sample sizes might cause some concern, even though credibility in qualitative research depends more on the richness of the information gathered (Patton, 1990). These sample sizes allowed for the collection of data of sufficient depth to address the aims of each study, and the key findings have also been reinforced by evidence from the wider literature.

Policy and Practice Implications

The findings of this research have a number of implications for public health practitioners, service providers and policy-makers seeking to address the growing issue of overweight and obesity. Feedback from participants regarding their reasons for seeking help highlights a range of ways to potentially increase recruitment to, and engagement with, weight loss interventions for specific client groups. For example, older adults and those with co-existing chronic illnesses are likely to respond best to recommendations and warnings from health professionals, whereas younger adults might respond to tailored promotional literature that encourages them to self-refer into programmes. Where services seek to recruit clients via professional recommendation, they must ensure that these professionals are fully aware of the aims of the service and that they feel confident in indentifying those who meet the eligibility criteria. The existing literature indicates a number of challenges that primary care practitioners experience in attempting to identify and manage overweight and obesity (Tod & Lacey, 2004). Research also suggests that health professionals may have negative attitudes towards these patients and that obese individuals may be reluctant to access services as a result (Alexander et al., 2006; Brown, 2006; Brown & Thompson, 2007; Richards et al., 2003). Training and support for practitioners can help to reduce the ambivalence or uneasiness they experience when measuring and discussing weight, which in turn should help to reduce ambivalence amongst clients and increase the likelihood of presentation with weight-related concerns. Assessing a client's readiness to change can also help to increase compliance with interventions and reduce the detrimental effects to others caused by poor retention rates. Programmes that intend to recruit participants by word of mouth and self-referral should consider adopting a social marketing approach in order to meet the needs and aspirations of their target audiences. In the case of Balance It, clients were involved in redesigning the programme's promotional literature in order to make it more appealing and accessible to those living in the target communities. They recommended the most suitable places to distribute the literature and were also keen to act as ambassadors for the programme, by helping to recruit and support future cohorts of clients. This type of peer-based approach has the potential to increase engagement with typically 'hard to reach' groups, enhance equity of service provision and ensure compliance with interventions (Donaldson, 2003; Lorig, 2002).

Rather than advocating a 'one-size-fits-all' approach, service providers must acknowledge that the most salient factors in the decision to lose weight vary by age, gender, health and family status. Ethnicity is likely to be an additional source of variation which has not been explored in our research due to the ethnic composition of the target populations. Our findings suggest that women are more likely than men to respond to messages relating to image factors. However, if the benefits for their appearance are used as arguments for encouraging weight loss, care must be taken not to increase the level of victimisation already felt by many obese individuals. A paradigm shift from weight-centred to health-centred approaches might help to reduce weight stigmatisation and also reduce the public's preoccupation with appearance (Barker & Cooke, 1992). This would require an additional shift in emphasis away from secondary and tertiary approaches to obesity treatment, towards primary prevention of excess weight in the general population. In the case of SWiMS, this Level 1 activity was conducted entirely separate from the Level 2 and 3 interventions, whereas it was part of the remit of the community-based Balance It programme. The perceived acceptability and effectiveness of both programmes suggests that a tiered approach to weight management can be successful, where interventions are tailored to the needs and preferences of client groups at different stages in the life cycle and at different points on the health/illness continuum. A primary care clinic was an appropriate venue for delivering the SWiMS programme because the clients all had co-morbidities that meant they were familiar with clinical health settings. The bottom-up approach of the Balance It intervention meant that the programme was delivered in venues identified as being suitable and accessible by members of the target communities. Participants in the social marketing research that informed the development of Balance It also requested opportunities to develop their cooking skills, which were valued most by those with young children and grandchildren. Women are still more likely than men to be involved in food purchasing and preparation, and therefore to find messages about ways to improve their family's health most appealing. By offering practical demonstrations and easy-to-prepare recipes, weight loss programmes may be able to have a wider impact on the health of their clients' families and their local communities.

Traditional nutritional education programmes tended to ignore the environmental impacts on health that are beyond an individual's immediate control, and therefore have the potential to widen rather than reduce inequalities (Freire, 1970). The holistic approaches of the interventions described here meant that it was possible to address these issues to some extent; for example, by teaching participants how to prepare local foods using healthy, affordable ingredients. It is crucial that service providers acknowledge the environmental constraints to individual behaviour change and the influence of the social context on people's health. This is particularly important for individuals living in areas of multiple deprivation, where the adoption of healthy behaviours may involve overcoming deep-rooted social and cultural norms, as well as their own beliefs, attitudes and intentions. Two key predictors of individual behaviour change are self-efficacy (a person's confidence that they can successfully change their behaviour) and outcome expectancy (a person's expectation that changing their behaviour will lead to the desired outcome) (Bandura, 1998). Linking these two principles is the idea that setting mini goals can help to improve an individual's sense of self-efficacy by providing markers of increasing mastery, evidenced here by reports of increased confidence after participants had successfully made and maintained small lifestyle changes. Similar interventions might benefit from incorporating advice around goal-setting and monitoring, in order to maintain motivation and enhance self-efficacy amongst clients. It is clear that a successful outcome is more likely where the benefits of behaviour change are perceived to outweigh the costs. Participants in our research reported finding the sessions more enjoyable than previous attempts to lose weight via commercial slimming groups or individual diet and exercise plans. The use of appropriate physical activity to complement nutritional education can result in tangible health and fitness improvements, which seem to reinforce the messages delivered and act as facilitators to further lifestyle changes. The existing literature also suggests that exercise increases dietary adherence and should therefore be seen as an integral part of any lifestyle intervention (Rodin & Plante, 1989). Walking tends to be the preferred form of activity, particularly for older and previously sedentary individuals. However, other options for taking part in activities at varying intensity levels should be offered at local venues and made affordable for those on low incomes.

The research described in this chapter suggests that overweight and obese individuals benefit from taking part in group education and activity sessions, but that they may need some assistance in overcoming initial feelings of fear or anxiety. As stated previously, allowing participants to attend sessions with a friend or family member can help to reduce this anxiety and also improve the outcomes of the intervention. Morbidly obese individuals and those who feel particularly self-conscious about their weight should be given the option of receiving one-to-one support, but the benefits of group support in terms of social interaction, developing new social networks and reducing isolation should be emphasised. Peers are also able to influence the behaviour of others because people are more likely to imitate a behaviour if a model appears to be a realistic figure for self-comparison (Pervin, 1989). It is known that messages are more likely to be accepted if they are delivered by someone similar to the audience but with greater prestige, if they are reinforced by the processes of peer pressure and support, and if the information they contain is useful, simply put, relevant, positive and novel (Foulger, 2004). Staff involved in delivering weight loss interventions must be friendly, approachable and understanding, but also knowledgeable about ways to tackle excess weight and skilled in translating this evidence into practice. Holistic interventions delivered by multi-disciplinary teams can inspire confidence amongst clients and continuity within the team allows for the development of trusting relationships with staff. Our participants emphasised the importance of providing opportunities for ongoing support from professionals and peers in order to maintain motivation, and supervision and surveillance are known to be important in preventing relapse amongst those who successfully lose weight (Sarlio-Lahteenkorva, 1998). Although peers can provide a degree of emotional support, they may be less well equipped than professionals to offer the necessary instrumental, informational and appraisal support required by overweight and obese individuals (House, 1981). Suggestions from our study participants included offering open groups rather than time-limited programmes, allowing drop-in access after completing the structured intervention, delivering occasional update meetings or one-off refresher sessions. Locating sessions in the community, rather than in health care settings, could help to facilitate client engagement with, and transition from, these weight loss programmes.

Recommendations for Future Research

The studies described in this chapter have added a depth of understanding to a complex public health issue. However, they also highlight the need for additional research to identify ways to successfully prevent, treat and manage overweight and obesity. The existing evidence on effective interventions for the prevention of weight gain and maintenance of weight loss continues to be of poorer quality compared with that for the treatment of obesity. A longer term follow-up of the study samples would allow for an exploration of the sustainability of the lifestyle changes made and identify the barriers or facilitators to participants' ongoing weight loss efforts. Further exploration with a larger sample of participants is also needed to investigate the factors that influence successful weight loss or regain amongst different target groups. For example, age, gender and ethnicity are known to influence weight-related beliefs and behaviours, and so it would be enlightening to investigate these variables more explicitly. There is also a need for research to gather the views of individuals who are overweight or obese but who do not access the available treatments and interventions for whatever reason. This is particularly the case for individuals living in disadvantaged communities or from marginalised, vulnerable or 'hidden' populations. Community- and population-based approaches may be the most effective method for halting the current trends in adult obesity, but the evidence to support this assumption is still lacking. It has been noted by previous authors that conventional studies in nutrition have tended to focus on the 'post-swallowing' world of biology, physiology, biochemistry and pathology, and neglected the 'pre-swallowing' domain of behaviour, culture, society and experience (Crotty, 1993; Germov & Williams, 1996). Qualitative research enables understanding of the range of different perspectives held by policy makers, service providers, practitioners and current or potential service users. This type of in-depth work is necessary to explore the social context of food and investigate the different meanings and understandings that emerge between places and individuals. A socio-ecological perspective, along with community-based participatory approaches to research and evaluation, may also help to shed light on the root causes of overweight and obesity.

Real world evaluation of weight loss interventions is inevitably challenging, as debate continues about what represents good practice in research and evaluation of health promotion (Millward et al., 2001). A balance is required between an outcomes-based approach that investigates efficacy and effectiveness, and qualitative approaches that examine processes of engagement, quality of interactions and user satisfaction. Also, more research tends to be devoted to the study of 'early successes' than to long-term maintenance of behaviour and lifestyle changes. It is therefore recommended that the concept of long-term maintenance should be redefined to allow for less-than-optimal goals, with both participants and service providers accepting more modest levels of achievement as indicators of success (Ory et al., 2002). Intermediate outcomes to be measured might include increases in knowledge of nutrition, self-reported physical activity levels and self-efficacy. However, these indicators should be locally defined with input from service users, practitioners and other key stakeholders in order to ensure their relevance within a particular context. They should also take into account changes in the wider determinants of health. In particular, it is recommended that the impact of community-based interventions be assessed across the breadth of their activities and settings, not just by changes in individual behaviour. The findings of this research highlight the importance of ongoing monitoring of interventions in order to demonstrate their short, medium and long-term implications for health and wellbeing. They also suggest a need for further research with practitioners involved in referring to such interventions, in order to identify perceived barriers and facilitators to successful recruitment or identification of clients. Key stakeholders, including service users, should be actively involved in the process of monitoring and evaluating interventions, and consulted at regular intervals to ensure their ongoing acceptability and suitability. Finally, it is important to devise and implement strategies for the wide dissemination of findings from successful weight loss interventions in order for others to learn from these examples of good practice.

ACKNOWLEDGMENTS

We would like to acknowledge the 'Balance It! It's Your Health' programme steering group and the Specialist Weight Management Service programme manager for their assistance in developing the study protocols and for overseeing the conduct of the research. The SWiMS evaluation was funded by Newcastle Primary Care Trust and the Balance It evaluation was funded by Gateshead Primary Care Trust on behalf of the programme steering group. Shelina Visram is currently funded by a Research Training Fellowship from the National Institute of Health Research (NIHR). Our colleagues Helen Cording and Lesley Geddes provided invaluable assistance with data collection during the original studies, and administrative support was provided by Yvonne Howard and Rosemary Reay at Northumbria

University. Finally, we would like to thank the clients of the SWiMS and Balance It programmes who gave up their time to participate in the interviews and focus groups.

References

Adolfsson, B., Carlson, A., Unden, A. & Rossner, S. (2002). Treating obesity: a qualitative evaluation of a lifestyle intervention for weight reduction. *Health Education Journal, 61(3),* 244-258.

Alexander, S., Ostbye, T., Pollack, K., Gradison, M., Bastian, L. & Namenek-Brouwer, R. (2006). Physicians' beliefs about discussing obesity: results from focus groups. *American Journal of Health Promotion, 21(6),* 498-500.

Allender, S. & Rayner, M. (2007). The burden of overweight and obesity-related ill health in the UK. *Obesity Reviews, 8(5)*, 467-473.

APHO. (2008a). *Health Profile 2008. North East*. Department of Health and the Association of Public Health Observatories: Accessed from www.healthprofiles.info.

APHO. (2008b). *Health Profile 2008. Newcastle upon Tyne*. Department of Health and the Association of Public Health Observatories: Accessed from www.healthprofiles.info.

APHO. (2008c). *Health Profile 2008. Gateshead*. Department of Health and the Association of Public Health Observatories: Accessed from www.healthprofiles.info.

Astrup, A., Grunwald, G., Melanson, E., Saris, W., & Hill, J. (2000). The role of low-fat diets in body weight control: a meta-analysis of ad libitum dietary intervention studies. *International Journal of Obesity 25*, 1545-1552.

Azjen, I. (1991). The theory of planned behaviour. *Organizational Behavior and Human Decision Processes 50*, 179-211.

Bandura, A. (1977). Self-efficacy: towards a unifying theory of behaviour change. *Psychological Review 84*, 191-215.

Bandura, A. (1997). *Self-efficacy: the exercise of control*. New York: Freeman.

Bandura, A. (1998). Health promotion from the perspective of Social Cognitive Theory. *Psychology & Health, 13*, 623-649.

Barker, R. & Cooke, B. (1992). Diet, obesity and being overweight: a qualitative research study. *Health Education Journal, 51(3),* 117-121.

Becker, E., Margraf, J., Turke, V., Soeder, U. & Neumer, S. (2001). Obesity and mental illness in a representative sample of young women. *International Journal of Obesity and Related Metabolic Disorders 25*(suppl. 1), S5-9.

Benner, P. (1994). *Interpretive Phenomenology: embodiment, caring, and ethics in health and illness*. Thousand Oaks, CA: Sage Publications.

Bidgood, J. & Buckroyd, J. (2005). An exploration of obese adults' experience of attempting to lose weight and to maintain a reduced weight. *Counselling and Psychotherapy Research, 5(3)*, 221-229.

Boslaugh, S. (2007). *Secondary Data Sources for Public Health. A Practical Guide*. Cambridge: Cambridge University Press.

Boyatzis, R. (1998). *Transforming Qualitative Information: thematic analysis and code development*. London: Sage.

Brown, I. (2006). Nurses' attitudes towards adult patients who are obese: literature review. *Journal of Advanced Nursing, 53(2),* 221-232.

Brown, I. & Thompson, J. (2007). Primary care nurses' attitudes, beliefs and own body size in relation to obesity management. *Journal of Advanced Nursing, 60(5),* 535-543.

Butland, B., Jebb, S., Kopelman, P., McPherson, K., Thomas, S., Mardell, J., et al. (2007). *Foresight. Tackling Obesities: Future Choices - Project report.* London: Government Office for Science.

Byrne, S. (2002). Psychological aspects of weight maintenance and relapse in obesity. *Journal of Psychosomatic Research, 53(5),* 1029-1036.

Byrne, S., Cooper, Z. & Fairburn, C. (2003). Weight maintenance and relapse in obesity: a qualitative study. *International Journal of Obesity, 27,* 955-962.

Campbell, R., Pound, P., Pope, C., Britten, N., Pill, R., Morgan, M., et al. (2003). Evaluating meta-ethnography: a synthesis of qualitative research on lay experiences of diabetes and diabetes care. *Social Science & Medicine, 56(4),* 671-684.

Carver, C. & Scheier, M. (1998). *On the Self-Regulation of Behaviour.* New York: Cambridge University Press.

Cioffi, J. (2002a). Clients' experiences of a weight management programme: a qualitative study. *Health Education 102(1),* 16-22.

Cioffi, J. (2002b). Factors that enable and inhibit transition from a weight management program: a qualitative study. *Health Education Research, 17(1),* 19-26.

Clark, M., Cargill, B., Medeiros, M. & Pera, V. (1996). Changes in self-efficacy following obesity treatment. *Obesity Research, 4,* 179-181.

Cording, H., Visram, S. & Crosland, A. (2005). *Evaluation of the Specialist Weight Management Service (SWiMS).* Newcastle-upon-Tyne: Northumbria University.

Cossrow, N., Jeffery, R. & McGuire, M. (2001). Understanding weight stigmatization: a focus group study. *Journal of Nutrition Education, 33,* 208-214.

Crotty, P. (1993). The value of qualitative research in nutrition. In *Annual Review of Health Social Science.* Deakin University: Centre for the Study of Body and Society.

Denzin, N. (1978). *The Research Act: a theoretical introduction to sociological methods. 2nd edition.* . New York: McGraw Hill.

Department of Health. (2004). *Choosing Health: making healthy choices easier.* London: Department of Health.

Despres, J., Lemieux, I. & Prud'homme, D. (2001). Treatment of obesity: need to focus on high risk abdominally obese patients. *BMJ, 322,* 716-720.

Donaldson, L. (2003). Expert patients usher in a new era of opportunity for the NHS. *BMJ, 326*(7402), 1279-1280.

Douglas, F., Greener, J. & Teijlingen, E. v. (2008). 'Ask me why I'm fat!' The need to engage with potential recipients of health promotion policy to prevent obesity. *The Australian Economic Review, 41(1),* 72-77.

DWP. (2008). *Effects of Obesity.* Department of Work and Pensions: Accessed from http://www.dwp.gov.uk/medical/med_conditions/obesity/effects_obesity.asp.

Ebbeling, C., Pawlak, D. & Ludwig, D. (2002). Childhood obesity: public-health crisis, common sense cure. *The Lancet, 360,* 473-482.

Effective Health Care. (1997). *The prevention and treatment of obesity. EHC Bulletin.* York: Centre for Reviews and Dissemination, University of York.

English, C. (1993). Gaining and losing weight: identity transformations. *Deviant Behaviour, 14*, 227-241.

Ensrud, K., Fullman, R., Barrett-Cooper, E., Cauley, J., Stefanick, M., Fink, H., et al. (2005). Voluntary weight reduction in older men increases hip bone loss: the osteoporotic fractures in men study. *Journal of Clinical Endocrinology and Metabolism, 90*, 1998-2004.

Epstein, L., Valoski, A., Wing, R. & McCurley, J. (1994). Ten year outcomes of behavioural family-based treatment of childhood obesity. *Health Psychology, 13*, 373-383.

Fielding, N. (1994). Varieties of research interviews. *Nurse Researcher, 1(3),* 4-13.

Foulger, D. (2004). *Models of the Communication Process.* . Evolutionary Media: Accessed from http://foulger.info/davis/research/unifiedModelOfCommunication.htm.

Freire, P. (1970). *Pedagogy of the Oppressed*. New York: Continuum.

Germov, J. & Williams, L. (1996). The epidemic of dieting women: the need for a sociological approach to food and nutrition. *Appetite, 27*, 97-108.

Grant, P. & Boersma, H. (2005). Making sense of being fat: a hermeneutic analysis of adults' explanations for obesity. *Counselling and Psychotherapy Research, 5(3),* 212-220.

Health Select Committee. (2004). *Obesity. Third Report of Session 2003-04. Volume I. Report, together with formal minutes*. London: The Stationery Office.

Heffernan, A. (2003). Obesity - a lifestyle issue. *World of Irish Nursing 11*, 37-39.

House, J. (1981). *Work Stress and Social Support*. Englewood Cliffs, NJ: Prentice Hall.

Institute of Nutrition Metabolism and Diabetes. (2003). Obesity in Canada. Identifying Policy Priorities.

Johnson, R. (1997). Examining the validity structure of qualitative research. *Education, 118(2),* 282-292.

Joint Health Surveys Unit. (2004). *Health Survey for England 2003*. London: Department of Health.

Jones, N., Furlanetto, D., Jackson, J. & Kinn, S. (2007). An investigation of obese adults' views of the outcomes of dietary treatment. *Journal of Human Nutrition and Dietetics, 20*, 486-494.

Jung, R. (1997). Obesity as a disease. *British Medical Bulletin 53*(2), 307-321.

Kayman, S., Bruvold, W. & Stern, J. (1990). Maintenance and relapse after weight loss in women: behavioural aspects. *American Journal of Clinical Nutrition, 52*, 800-807.

Kopelman, P. (2000). Obesity as a medical problem. *Nature, 404*, 635-643.

Kreuger, R. (1988). *Focus Groups: A Practical Guide for Applied Research*. London: Sage.

Lavery, M. & Loewy, K. (1993). Identifying predictive variables for long term weight change after participation in a weight loss program. *Journal of the American Dietetic Association, 93*, 1017-1024.

Lean, M., Han, T. & Morrison, C. (1995). Waist circumference as a measure for indicating need for weight management. *BMJ, 311*, 158-161.

Lemieux, S., Prud'homme, D., Bouchard, C., Tremblay, A. & Després, J. (1996a). A single threshold value of waist girth identifies normal-weight and overweight subjects with excess visceral adipose tissue. *American Journal of Clinical Nutrition 64*, 685-693.

Lemieux, S., Prud'homme, D., Tremblay, A., Bouchard, C. & Despres, J. (1996b). Anthropometric correlates to changes in visceral adipose tissue over 7 years in women. *International Journal of Obesity and Related Metabolic Disorders, 20*, 618-624.

Lincoln, Y. & Guba, E. (1985). *Naturalistic Inquiry* Beverly Hills, CA: Sage.

Lorig, K. (2002). Partnerships between expert patients and physicians. *Lancet, 359*(9309), 814-815.

Marcus, B., Eaton, C., Rossi, J. & Harlow, L. (1994). Self-efficacy, decision making and stages of change: an integrative model of physical exercise. *Journal of Applied Social Psychology 24*, 489-508.

Marcus, B. & Owen, N. (1992). Motivational readiness, self-efficacy and decision making for exercise. *Journal of Applied Social Psychology 22*, 3-16.

Marcus, B., Rossi, J., Selby, V., Niaura, R. & Abrams, D. (1992). Self-efficacy and the stages of exercise behaviour change. *Research Quarterly for Exercise and Sport, 63*, 60-66.

Millward, L., Kelly, M. & Nutbeam, D. (2001). *Public health intervention research: the evidence*. London: Health Development Agency.

Morgan, D. (1997). *Focus Groups as Qualitative Research. 2nd edition*. London: Sage.

Mulvihill, C. & Quigley, R. (2003). *The management of obesity and overweight: an analysis of reviews of diet, physical activity and behavioural approaches*. London: Health Development Agency.

National Audit Office. (2001). *Tackling Obesity in England*. London: The Stationery Office.

National Heart Lung and Blood Institute. (1998). *Clinical guidelines on the identification, evaluation and treatment of overweight and obesity in adults. The evidence report.* Bethseda, MD: National Institutes of Health.

NEPHO. (2007). *Occasional Paper No. 28. Obesity: A North East Update Report.* . Stockton-on-Tees: North East Public Health Observatory.

Newman, A., Yanez, D., Harris, T., Duxbury, A., Enright, P. & Fried, L. (2001). Weight change in old age and its association with mortality. *Journal of the American Geriatric Society, 49*, 1309-1318.

NHS Centre for Reviews and Dissemination. (1997). *A systematic review of the interventions for the prevention and treatment of obesity, and the maintenance of weight loss. CRD Report 10*. York: Centre for Reviews and Dissemination, University of York

NICE. (2006). *Obesity: the prevention, identification, assessment and management of overweight and obesity in adults and children*. London: National Institute for Health and Clinical Excellence.

NICE. (2007). *Behaviour change at population, community and individual levels*. London: National Institute for Health and Clinical Excellence

Noblit, G. & Hare, D. (1988). *Meta-Ethnography: Synthesizing Qualitative Studies*. London: Sage.

Ory, M. G., Jordan, P. J. & Bazzarre, T. (2002). The Behaviour Change Consortium: setting the stage for a new century of health behaviour-change research. *Health Education Research, 17*, 500-511.

Parham, E. (1993). Enhancing social support in weight loss management groups. *Journal of the American Dietetic Association, 93*(10), 1152-1156.

Patton, M. (1990). *Qualitative Evaluation and Research Methods. 2nd edition*. Newbury Park, CA: Sage Publications.

Pervin, L. A. (1989). *Personality: Theory and Research* (5th edition ed.). New York: Wiley.

Pirozzo, S., Sumerbell, C., Cameron, C. & Glasziou, P. (2002). Advice on low-fat diets for obesity. *Cochrane Database of Systematic Reviews, 2*(CD003640).

Popay, J. & Williams, G. (1996). Public health research and lay knowledge. *Social Science & Medicine, 42*(5), 759-768.

Prochaska, J. & DiClemente, C. (1986). Toward a comprehensive model of change. In W. Miller & N. Heather (Eds.), *Addictive Behaviors: Processes of Change* (pp. 3-27). New York: Plenum Press.

Prospective Studies Collaboration. (2009). Body-mass index and cause-specific mortality in 900,000 adulta: collaborative analyses of 57 prospective studies. *The Lancet, 373*(9669), 1083-1096.

Reilly, J., Wilson, M., Summerbell, C. & Wilson, D. (2002). Obesity: diagnosis, prevention, and treatment; evidence based answers to common questions. *Archives of Disease in Childhood, 86*, 392-395.

Richards, H., Reid, M. & Watt, G. (2003). Victim-blaming revisited: a qualitative study of beliefs about illness causation, and responses to chest pain. *Family Practice, 20(6),* 711-716.

Roberts, A. & Ashley, G. (1999). What are the characteristics of overweight and obese patients who achieve weight loss and what factors are most helpful? A quantitative and qualitative study of patients in a rural general practice. *Journal of Human Nutrition and Dietetics, 12*(suppl. 1), 20-27.

Robson, C. (2002). *Real World Research*. Oxford: Blackwell.

Rodin, J. & Plante, T. (1989). The psychological effects of exercise. In R. Williams & A. Wallace (Eds.), *Biological Effects of Physical Activity* (pp. 127-136). Champaign, IL: Human Kinetics.

Rogge, M., Greenwald, M. & Golden, A. (2004). Obesity, stigma, and civilized oppression. *Advances in Nursing Science, 27(4),* 301-315.

Rollnick, S., Kinnersley, P. & Stott, N. (1993). Methods of helping patients with behaviour change. *BMJ, 307*, 188-190.

Sallis, J., Haskell, W., Fortmann, S., Vranizan, K., Taylor, C. & Solomon, D. (1986). Predictors of adoption and maintenance of physical activity in a community sample. *Preventive Medicine 15*, 331-341.

Sarlio-Lahteenkorva, S. (1998). Relapse stories in obesity. *European Journal of Public Health, 8*, 203-209.

Sarlio-Lahteenkorva, S. (2000). 'The battle is not over after weight loss': stories of successful weight maintenance. *Health, 4(1),* 73-88.

Seefeldt, V., Malina, R. & Clark, M. (2002). Factors affecting levels of physical activity in adults. *Sports Medicine, 32(3),* 143-168.

SMS. (2004). *A Local Baseline Study of Body Mass Index*. Newcastle-upon-Tyne: Survey & Marketing Services Ltd.

SMS. (2006). *An investigation into attitudes and perceptions of weight and weight loss*. Newcastle-upon-Tyne: Survey & Marketing Services Ltd.

The Health and Social Care Information Centre. (2009). *Statistics on obesity, physical activity and diet: England, February 2009*. Leeds: The NHS Information Centre.

Thomas, S., Hyde, J., Karunaratne, A., Herbert, D. & Komesaroff, P. (2008). Being 'fat' in today's world: a qualitative study of the lived experiences of people with obesity in Australia. *Health Expectations, 11*, 321-330.

Tod, A. & Lacey, A. (2004). Overweight and obesity: helping clients take action. *British Journal of Community Nursing, 9*(2), 59-66.

Troiano, R. & Flegel, K. (1998). Overweight children and adolescents: description, epidemiology and demographics. *Pediatrics 101*(suppl. 3), 497-504.

Visram, S., Crosland, A. & Cording, H. (in press). Triggers for weight gain and weight loss amongst patients of a primary care-based intervention: an exploratory study. *British Journal of Community Nursing*, in press.

Visram, S. & Geddes, L. (2007). *Evaluation of 'Balance It! It's Your Health' - A Programme to Reduce Adult Obesity / BMI in Gateshead. Final Report*. Newcastle-upon-Tyne: Northumbria University.

Visvanathan, R. & Chapman, I. (2005). Prognosis in obesity. Older people should not be misinformed about being overweight. *BMJ, 331*(7514), 452.

Wanless, D. (2004). *Securing Good Health for the Whole Population. Final report*. London: HM Treasury.

Wannamethee, S., Shaper, A. & Lennon, L. (2005). Reasons for intentional weight loss, unintentional weight loss, and mortality in older men. *Archives of Internal Medicine, 165*, 1035-1040.

Whitaker, R., Wright, J., Pepe, M., Seidel, K. & Dietz, W. (1997). Predicting obesity in young adulthood from childhood and parental obesity. *New England Journal of Medicine, 337*, 869-873.

WHO. (2000). Global database on Body Mass Index. Geneva: World Health Organisation:

WHO. (2004). *Global strategy on diet, physical activity and health*. Geneva: World Health Organisation. Accessed from http://www.who.int/dietphysicalactivity/publications/facts/obesity/en/

Wing, R. & Jeffery, R. (1999). Benefits of recruiting participants with friends and increasing social support for weight loss and maintenance. *Journal of Consulting and Clinical Psychology, 1*, 132-138.

In: Nutritional Education
Editor: Ida R. Laidyth

ISBN: 978-1-60876-078-7

Chapter 2

NUTRITION EDUCATION IN THE WORKPLACE: IMPACT ON DIET AND HEALTH

***A. D. Hutchinson*[1, 2], *B. Wilson*[1, 2] *and C. Wilson*[1, 2]**
1Flinders University, South Australia, Australia
2Cancer Council South Australia, Australia

ABSTRACT

Nutrition education programs have been implemented in the workplace in an effort to improve the diet and lifestyle of employees and, therefore, reduce the incidence of many chronic diseases linked to overweight and obesity including, diabetes, cardiovascular disease and cancer. Despite the importance of this outcome, the success of these programs has varied. This chapter uses a qualitative, narrative approach to review research conducted over the past 10 years on nutrition programs in the workplace and attempts to identify those aspects associated with successful behaviour change among employees. This approach enables us to include a variety of methods of intervention and data collection and thereby allows identification of promising intervention approaches that might not be identified in review approaches that are based on quantitative meta-analyses.

The chapter reviews the evidence for both the efficacy and the effectiveness of nutrition education programs in the workplace (i.e., whether an intervention works under ideal, well controlled conditions, versus whether the intervention works in the "uncontrolled" real-world workplace) (Spraycar, 1995). In addition, the characteristics of efficacious and effective programs are described including the duration of the nutrition education programs, the type of programs offered to employees, and the settings in which the programs were implemented. The results of the review suggest the workplace is a viable context for delivery of programs designed to change food intake behaviours, and overweight and obesity prevalence, although the challenge is to achieve sustained change on these outcomes after the intervention concludes. The results of this review should be taken into account when planning future work-based education programs on nutrition.

INTRODUCTION

Overweight and obesity are associated with an increased risk of many chronic diseases including cancer, cardiovascular disease, and diabetes (Kumanyika et al., 2008; McMillan, Sattar, & McArdle, 2006; Must et al., 1999). Consequently, obesity is associated with significant health and financial costs for individuals and the community. Behavioural treatments, including nutrition education designed to facilitate dietary change, have been shown to result in weight loss and prevention of weight gain.

The context in which these programs are delivered has varied with a range of different nutrition interventions rolled-out in schools, church groups, community settings and workplaces. In the workplace context, the motivation to tackle rates of overweight and obesity and associated chronic illness include; decreasing rates of absenteeism and sick leave, improving occupational health and safety outcomes, enhancing job satisfaction and organisational commitment, and decreasing staff turnover. In Britain, the National Audit Office (2004) estimated that obesity accounted for 18 million days of sickness absence and 18,000 premature deaths in 1998. Wanjek (2005) has argued that, in Canada, every $1.00 spent on workplace health promotion programs achieves cost savings through reduced sick days and increased productivity of between US$1.50 and US$5.75. Another study that has explored the potential financial savings of eight nutrition interventions reported that all were cost-effective because of the health benefits that flowed from the dietary changes achieved and the subsequent reduction in health expenditure (Dalziel & Segal, 2007).

The nature of the nutrition education programs that have been conducted and evaluated during the last decade has varied widely on dimensions that include sample size, type of intervention, duration of the intervention, the specific outcomes measured and the extent to which long term follow-up of treatment effects was conducted. As a consequence of the heterogeneity of these studies, the efficacy and effectiveness of nutrition interventions for overweight and obesity prevention or remediation remains unclear. The current chapter aims to review the research studies that have evaluated nutrition education programs in the workplace over the past 10 years.

The current review is limited to published studies and is therefore susceptible to the "file drawer problem" (Rosenthal, 1995). This refers to the tendency for studies with statistically significant results to be more likely to be published than studies with nonsignificant findings. Therefore, studies with nonsignificant results may be unreported and consequently excluded from reviews. However, the different approaches to nutrition education included in this review should be equally affected by this bias. Therefore, if one approach is more successful than another it is more likely to reflect the increased efficacy of the nutrition education program than a failure to include unpublished studies.

METHOD

The PubMed database was searched on the 17th of January 2009, using the terms (work or workplace or worksite) and (intervention or program) and (diet or nutrition or weight) in order to capture all potentially relevant studies. This search was limited to studies published in English between 1999 and 2008 and research involving human participants. A total of 1091 study references were identified using these criteria. Of these, 43 included a nutrition education program in the workplace, included healthy individuals (as opposed to targeting already unhealthy or high-risk employees), provided an evaluation of the program over time (i.e., not baseline data alone), and examined nutrition or health outcomes. Consequently, the studies reported here were repeated measures, controlled trials, unless otherwise reported in the results. An additional 5 studies were identified as part of a larger review that included exercise interventions in the workplace. Although nutrition was not the primary focus of these interventions, nutrition education was a significant component of the programs. Therefore, 48 studies were included in this review.

The results of these studies are summarised in Table 1. A description of the participants, the country in which the study took place and the number of participants in the study, including controls, is included in Table 1. In addition, whether participation was compulsory for all employees or voluntary is specified under population, for studies that provided this information. The duration of the intervention, and whether a post-test was conducted at the end of the intervention are also indicated. In the table of results, maintenance reflects the maintenance of any effects observed at the end of the intervention at a later follow-up period. For example, three months would indicate that an evaluation of the program was conducted at the end of the intervention and three months after the end of the intervention. The results reported were statistically significant unless indicated otherwise in Table 1.

RESULTS AND DISCUSSION

Approaches to Nutrition Education – What works?

The nutrition education undertaken in the studies in this review included a number of different approaches; seminars, health screening, individual counselling, web-based nutrition education, workplace nutrition changes and peer-based interventions. Health screening or medical examinations were incorporated into a number of the health promotion programs providing the opportunity to monitor biological and physiological indices of health, specifically, BMI, blood pressure, and cholesterol (Aldana, et al., 2002; Braeckman, et al., 1999; Gordon, et al., 2001; Prior et al., 2005; Renaud, et al., 2008; Talvi, et al., 1999; Williams, et al., 2004). This approach, although potentially expensive, allows objective health indicators to be obtained. The inclusion of biological markers of health is useful, particularly if the health assessments can be integrated into existing workplace practices, although their utility is likely to be poor where the intervention is minimal or the duration short. Under these circumstances, significant effects are unlikely to be observed. Other studies focused on self-report measures of attitudes, perceptions, knowledge, and behaviour, including dietary choices.

Several health promotion programs included individual counselling in their interventions (Atlantis, et al., 2006; Braeckman, et al., 1999; Elliot, et al., 2004; Moy, et al., 2006; Proper, et al., 2003; Sorensen, et al., 2007; Talvi, et al., 1999). Individual counselling allows nutrition advice to be tailored to the individual's needs and usually identifies barriers to dietary change. The aim of the counselling was generally described as setting behavioural goals that were specific to the individual. The advantage of this sort of approach is that it makes the intervention personally salient although the costs are high in time and money.

Web-based interventions have also been utilized to provide tailored nutrition recommendations and feedback (Block et al., 2004; Brug, 1999; Campbell et al., 2002; R. F. Cook et al., 2007; Cousineau et al., 2008; De Bourdeaudhuij et al., 2007; Papadaki & Scott, 2008; Petersen et al., 2008). These programs collect information from individual participants and then provide targeted advice for the individual based on the information provided. Web-based nutrition education programs have been shown to decrease dietary intake of fat, junk foods, pre-packaged foods and increase intake of fruits and vegetables, fish, whole grains, and water (Block et al., 2004; Brug, 1999; Campbell et al., 2002; De Bourdeaudhuij et al., 2007; Papadaki & Scott, 2008; Petersen et al., 2008). In addition, they have been shown to increase knowledge about nutrition, improve attitudes towards healthy eating, and reduce weight and cholesterol (R. F. Cook et al., 2007; Cousineau et al., 2008; Papadaki & Scott, 2008; Petersen et al., 2008). However, only two of these studies evaluated the outcomes after the intervention ended (Papadaki & Scott, 2008; Petersen et al., 2008) and only three studies compared a web-based delivery with alternative interventions (Brug, 1999; R. F. Cook et al., 2007; Papadaki & Scott, 2008).

Web-based programs present a number of distinct advantages. They mimic the tailored advice provided through counselling in a cost-effective manner. They are also widely accessible and do not limit participation to workers in the same physical location. Therefore, these approaches would be suited to workers distributed across different cities or countries, those located in rural areas and those who work from home. In addition, many more traditional programs have supplemented education seminars or activities with emails, online newsletters, or health promotion websites to disseminate information (Plotnikoff et al., 2005; Polacsek et al., 2006).

Peer education programs utilise a less formal method for spreading nutrition messages. This approach identifies key individuals who disseminate the health promotion message by undertaking informal conversations with their peers. These peer educators, like web-based programs, are able to provide tailored nutrition information and advice but are also able to lead by example and take advantage of existing social networks. The Arizona 5-a-day Peer Education Program utilized this approach and found that the program led to increased consumption of fruits, vegetables, and juices and that these changes were associated with contact with peer educators (Buller et al., 2000; Buller et al., 1999). Although most of the dietary changes were no longer significant 6 months after the program's conclusion, positive changes in nutrition knowledge and diet-related attitudes persisted at the 6 month follow-up.

The Coronary Heart Improvement Project, evaluated by Aldana et al. (2005), was among the most effective interventions in that it not only achieved dietary change but these changes translated into a significant reduction in BMI in employees over a six-month period. The Coronary Heart Improvement Project included education sessions on a range of topics including obesity, coronary heart risks, cancer, diet, exercise, behaviour change, and self-worth. It also incorporated input from dieticians and medical professionals, utilized textbooks and workbooks, and contained practical skills training during tours of supermarkets and cooking demonstrations. Although this intervention did not use a particularly innovative approach, it was a comprehensive and well planned program.

Table 1. Results from health promotion interventions, including nutrition education programs

REFERENCE	POPULATION (Sample, Country, *N*, recruitment)	INTERVENTION	DURATION	POST-TEST	MAINTENANCE	RESULTS	COMMENTS
(Block et al., 2008)	Employees of a health care organization U.S.A. 787 participants (549 at post-test) Voluntary participation	Email intervention Individualized feedback, goals, reminders and promotion of social support Targets: increasing physical activity, intake of fruits and vegetables, and decreasing dietary fats and sugars	4 months	✓	×	Improvement in stage of change for fats and fruits and vegetables, self-efficacy for dietary change	Dietary changes not measured
(Chen, Wu, & Gu, 2008)	Steel factory employees China 110, 000 employees	Set-up health networks, health education and promotion, and training for health professionals Targets: moderate drinking, overweight and obesity, nutrition (reduced salt and fat content) along with smoking cessation, and physical activity	9 years	✓	×	↓ salt intake, diastolic blood pressure	Fat intake not reported

Note: Maintenance period refers to the time of evaluation in terms of the number of weeks or months after the intervention finished

Table 1. (Continued)

REFERENCE	POPULATION (Sample, Country, *N*, recruitment)	INTERVENTION	DURATION	POST-TEST	MAINTENANCE	RESULTS	COMMENTS
(Cousineau, Houle, Bromberg, Fernandez, & Kling, 2008)	Gaming establishment employees U.S.A. 54 employees Voluntary participation	Tailored nutrition web program (*Working on My Health: Nutrition*) Nutrition assessment, information and strategies	30 minutes	✓	✗	↑ in nutrition knowledge	No control group Prototype of program
(Papadaki & Scott, 2008)	22-55 y.o. female, university employees Scotland 72 employees Voluntary participation	Tailored dietary feedback and goal setting, internet education (Mediterranean eating website) vs. minimal dietary feedback and general nutrition brochures	6 months	✓	3 months	Post-test: ↑ fruits, nuts, seeds, vegetables ↑ HDL cholesterol ↓ total:HDL cholesterol ratio Maintenance at 3 months: ↑ vegetables ↑ HDL cholesterol ↓ total:HDL cholesterol ratio	

Note: Maintenance period refers to the time of evaluation in terms of the number of weeks or months after the intervention finished

Table 1. (Continued)

REFERENCE	POPULATION (Sample, Country, *N*, recruitment)	INTERVENTION	DURATION	POST-TEST	MAINTENANCE	RESULTS	COMMENTS
(Petersen, Sill, Lu, Young, & Edington, 2008)	IBM employees U.S.A. 7743 employees (1639 at 6 months follow-up) Voluntary participation	Interactive online weight management program (Virtual Food Pro) Targets included dietary habits and physical activity	Self-paced	No distinct end point because the program was self-paced	6 months 12 months	↓ weight ↓ junk food, fast food, pre-packaged food, dessert, and non-fast food restaurants ↑ fish, whole grains, water, fruit, legumes, vegetables, and dairy ↑ eating breakfast and taking lunch to work No significant difference in weight but significantly more in normal weight range in the intervention group	No control group Control group
(Renaud et al., 2008)	Employees of a financial organisation Canada 270 employees Voluntary participation	Take care of your health! program Educational sessions, health status profiles, voluntary telephone follow-up interviews Targets: global health, stress management, heart health, healthy eating and physical activity	3 years	✓	✗	↑ healthy eating habits e.g. 3 serves of fruits or fruit juices, 3 serves of vegetables or vegetable juices, eating whole-grain cereal products every day, limiting fat intake 34% reported losing weight	No control group

Note: Maintenance period refers to the time of evaluation in terms of the number of weeks or months after the intervention finished

Table 1. (Continued)

REFERENCE	POPULATION (Sample, Country, *N*, recruitment)	INTERVENTION	DURATION	POST-TEST	MAINTENANCE	RESULTS	COMMENTS
(R. F. Cook, Billings, Hersch, Back, & Hendrickson, 2007)	Human resources company employees U.S.A. 480 employees (419 at post-test) Voluntary participation	Web-based multimedia health promotion: diet, stress, and PA vs. print health promotion	3 months	✓	✗	No difference between the groups except the web-based intervention had greater improvement on attitudes toward a healthful diet and dietary stage of change Both groups showed improvements in diet and achieved a small amount of weight loss (pre-post within group comparisons)	NB: comparison with print rather than no intervention
(De Bourdeaudhuij, Stevens, Vandelanotte, & Brug, 2007)	Employees of companies that showed interest Belgium 539 employees (337 at 6 month follow-up)	Fat intake program Interactive computer tailored intervention vs. generic intervention (non-tailored advice) vs. no intervention	Not specified	✓ (6 months after baseline)	✗	↓ fat intake	

Note: Maintenance period refers to the time of evaluation in terms of the number of weeks or months after the intervention finished

Table 1. (Continued)

REFERENCE	POPULATION (Sample, Country, *N*, recruitment)	INTERVENTION	DURATION	POST-TEST	MAINTENANCE	RESULTS	COMMENTS
(Sorensen et al., 2007) & (Sorensen et al., 2005)	Employees from small businesses that employed a multi-ethnic workforce U.S.A. 974 employees (completing baseline and follow-up) Voluntary participation	Healthy directions small business study Targeted to each worksite Individual behaviour change, environmental support, and organisational change Targets: healthy eating, physical activity, smoking cessation and reduction of hazardous occupational exposures	18 months	✓	✗	↑ Multivitamin use ↑ fruit and vegetable consumption was associated with supportive social norms, food sufficiency, and strong social networks	
(Atlantis, Chow, Kirby, & Fiatarone Singh, 2006)	Casino employees Australia 73 employees (42 at post-test) Voluntary participation	Supervised exercise program Behaviour modification strategies (group seminars, one-on-one counselling, worksite manual) Dietary component: encouraged to decrease servings of energy dense foods,	24 weeks	✓	✗	↓ waist circumference No change in BMI No results given for dietary changes	

Note: Maintenance period refers to the time of evaluation in terms of the number of weeks or months after the intervention finished

Table 1. (Continued)

REFERENCE	POPULATION (Sample, Country, *N*, recruitment)	INTERVENTION	DURATION	POST-TEST	MAINTENANCE	RESULTS	COMMENTS
(Engbers, van Poppel, Chin, & van Mechelen, 2006)	Government office workers with a BMI>23 Netherlands 515 employees (432 at post-test) Voluntary participation	FoodSteps Intervention Food intervention: information sheets near food in the canteen, information on vending machines, information stand on healthy food, blood pressure, and cholesterol. The energy value of foods was translated into the number of minutes to burn this energy. Focus on food (healthy food choices) and physical activity	12 months	✓	×	¼ of the way through (3 months from baseline): Intervention led to more perceived social support in eating less fat No significant effect on fruit, vegetable, and fat intake Post-test: As above	
(Moy, Sallam, & Wong, 2006)	Male security guards working at a public university Malaysia 186 employees (150 at post-test) Voluntary participation	One to one counselling at least twice a year, group teaching 3-4 times a year, supportive environment Dietary advice was based on the National Cholesterol Education Programme (NCEP) Step 1 diet and the American Heart Association guide for cardiovascular health	24 months	✓	×	↓ cholesterol No change in BMI, blood pressure, glucose No significant differences in dietary measures	

Note: Maintenance period refers to the time of evaluation in terms of the number of weeks or months after the intervention finished

Table 1. (Continued)

REFERENCE	POPULATION (Sample, Country, *N*, recruitment)	INTERVENTION	DURATION	POST-TEST	MAINTENANCE	RESULTS	COMMENTS
(Polacsek, O'Brien, Lagasse, & Hammar, 2006)	Worksite and community based intervention U.S.A. 1860 employees Voluntary participation	Move & Improve Various forms of communication (e.g. newspaper, online newsletter) including information on nutrition Focus on physical activity	12 weeks	✓	×	Substantial proportion of participants reported ↓ weight, fat intake, television viewing, sugar-sweetened soft drink consumption, stress and ↑ intake of fruit and vegetables, energy, and water intake. Significance not reported.	Primarily a physical activity intervention Worksite and community based intervention
(Yancey et al., 2006)	Organisations, businesses and agencies in target areas of LA (staff, members, and clients) Targeted African Americans and Latinos U.S.A. 565 employees	Cardiovascular disease prevention Diabetes prevention Exercise breaks and lectures and discussions on: goal setting and motivation, nutrition, physical activity/fitness	12 weeks	✓	×	↑ intake of fruit and vegetables ↓ feelings of sadness or depression Trend ↓ BMI ($p = .08$)	No control group

Note: Maintenance period refers to the time of evaluation in terms of the number of weeks or months after the intervention finished

Table 1. (Continued)

REFERENCE	POPULATION (Sample, Country, *N*, recruitment)	INTERVENTION	DURATION	POST-TEST	MAINTENANCE	RESULTS	COMMENTS
(Aldana et al., 2005)	Medical care provider employees U.S.A. 145 employees (137 at 5 month maintenance period) Voluntary participation	Coronary Heart Improvement Project Education on health, diet, exercise, and behaviour change Input from dieticians, medical professionals, a textbook, workbooks, assignments, shopping tours and cooking demonstrations	4 weeks	not specified	2 weeks (6 weeks from baseline) 5 months (6 months from baseline)	↓ calories from fat ↑ carbohydrates, fruit and veg ↓ BMI, weight, cholesterol ↓ calories from fat, fat intake, dietary cholesterol, protein, servings of meat ↑ carbohydrates, fruits and vegetables ↓ BMI, weight	
(Plotnikoff, McCargar, Wilson, & Loucaides, 2005)	Employees from 3 government and 2 private sector organisations Canada 2121 employees Voluntary participation	Weekly emails with physical activity and nutrition messages Nutrition information: balance, variety and moderation, reducing fat intake, increasing fruit and vegetable intake	3 months	(see maintenance)	1 week (post-intervention)	Intervention group reported increased healthy eating practices, improved balance between food intake and physical activity, cooking meals with techniques to reduce fat and avoiding high-fat foods	

Note: Maintenance period refers to the time of evaluation in terms of the number of weeks or months after the intervention finished

Table 1. (Continued)

REFERENCE	POPULATION (Sample, Country, *N*, recruitment)	INTERVENTION	DURATION	POST-TEST	MAINTENANCE	RESULTS	COMMENTS
(Prior et al., 2005)	Employees from 162 companies Switzerland 4198 employees Voluntary participation	Reduction of cardiovascular risk factors Mobile unit Health screening, cardiovascular risk assessment, counselling if mildly elevated risk factors	15 mins	NA (see maintenance)	3.7 years (on average because different companies had different maintenance periods)	↓ diastolic blood pressure ↑ BMI, body weight ↑ cholesterol in women and no change in men	Very brief intervention No specific nutrition education described
(Block, Block, Wakimoto, & Block, 2004)	Corporate worksite employees U.S.A. 84 employees (47 at post-test) Voluntary participation	Worksite Internet Nutrition (WIN) Tailored to the individual Choice between reducing fat or increasing fruit and vegetables Skill facilitation, goal setting, reminders and reinforcement Family participation and support, information, social networks (bulletin board) and links to websites	12 weeks	✓	×	↓ dietary fat ↑ fruits and vegetables	Only 56% participated in the evaluation at the end of the program Results remained significant when a change score of 0 was assigned to non-responders

Note: Maintenance period refers to the time of evaluation in terms of the number of weeks or months after the intervention finished

Table 1. (Continued)

REFERENCE	POPULATION (Sample, Country, *N*, recruitment)	INTERVENTION	DURATION	POST-TEST	MAINTENANCE	RESULTS	COMMENTS
(Elliot et al., 2004)	Professional firefighters U.S.A. 33 firefighters	Promoting Healthy Lifestyles: Alternative Models' Effects (PHLAME) Team based intervention vs. client centred (individual meetings with trained health counsellor) vs. control Increase servings of fruit and veg, physical activity, energy balance, reduce fat intake and normalize body fat	6 months	✓	✗	Both interventions: ↓ LDL cholesterol Team: ↑ coworker cohesion, personal exercise habits, coworkers' healthy behaviours One-on-one: ↑ dietary self-monitoring, ↓ fat intake, depressed feelings	
(Gill & Wijk, 2004)	Professional drivers passing through truck stops Sweden 120 drivers Voluntary participation	National healthy eating intervention Information campaign Offering healthy food choice alternatives Menu changes (presentation and content) Truck stop food content Training of staff Incentives for healthy choices	3 years	✓	✗	↑ nutritional awareness ↑ in healthier food choices by drivers (qualitative data) Specials were more balanced in terms of fat, calories, carbohydrates and protein content	No control group Evaluation was conducted using interviews, field observations, and questionnaires

Note: Maintenance period refers to the time of evaluation in terms of the number of weeks or months after the intervention finished

Table 1. (Continued)

REFERENCE	POPULATION (Sample, Country, *N*, recruitment)	INTERVENTION	DURATION	POST-TEST	MAINTENANCE	RESULTS	COMMENTS
(Holdsworth, Raymond, & Haslam, 2004)	Employees from various workplaces England 1153 employees (577 at post-test)	Heartbeat Award scheme Information, reminders and reinforcement for behaviour change Supportive environment Nutrition goals: reduce fat, sugar and salt and increase fibre-rich, starchy foods	6 months	✓	✗	Significantly more positive change in 4 out of 20 foods tested: ↑ fruit, ↓ fried food and sweet puddings, and change to low fat milk	Baseline data was taken 6 months prior to the Heartbeat Award scheme
(Shimizu, Horiguchi, Kato, & Nagata, 2004)	Employees from manufacturing companies Japan 629 employees	Health interviews, measurements and group education on nutrition, exercise and stress management	4 years	✓	✗	↓ BMI and systolic blood pressure in under 35 year olds ↓ Serum total cholesterol, HDL cholesterol in over 35 year olds	

Note: Maintenance period refers to the time of evaluation in terms of the number of weeks or months after the intervention finished

Table 1. (Continued)

REFERENCE	POPULATION (Sample, Country, *N*, recruitment)	INTERVENTION	DURATION	POST-TEST	MAINTENANCE	RESULTS	COMMENTS
(Steenhuis et al., 2004)	Employees (mostly white collar) from large Dutch companies The Netherlands 1013 respondents (completed both pre and post-test)	Cafeteria interventions Compared an educational program (eating less fat, more fruits and vegetables) a food supply program (increased availability of healthy foods), a labelling program (labelling of low fat products) and a control group (no program) Fat, fruit and vegetable intake	4 weeks	✓	✗	Labelling program led to ↓ fat intake for participants who believed they ate a high fat diet and ↑ sales of low fat desserts	
(Williams, Wold, Dunkin, Idleman, & Jackson, 2004)	Low-income African American female employees at urban and rural worksites U.S.A. 294 employees Voluntary participation	Diet and physical activity Behaviour change to reduce risk of cardiovascular disease	not specified	✓	✗	↓ % with elevated cholesterol ↓ dietary fat intake in rural women	No control group

Note: Maintenance period refers to the time of evaluation in terms of the number of weeks or months after the intervention finished

Table 1. (Continued)

REFERENCE	POPULATION (Sample, Country, *N*, recruitment)	INTERVENTION	DURATION	POST-TEST	MAINTENANCE	RESULTS	COMMENTS
(Abood, Black, & Feral, 2003)	University employees U.S.A. 33 employees Voluntary participation	Nutrition education program Weekly 1 hour education sessions from a dietician for 8 weeks Promotion of knowledge and beliefs to improve diet Tailored by baseline assessments and addressed perceived benefits and barriers	8 weeks	✓	✗	↑ perceived benefits of positive dietary behaviours ↑ knowledge about nutrition and CVD and cancer prevention ↓ energy intake, fat and cholesterol intake	
(Proper, Hildebrandt, Van der Beek, Twisk, & Van Mechelen, 2003)	Employees from municipal services The Netherlands 299 employees Voluntary participation	Individual counselling on physical activity, fitness and health Content derived from the Patient-centred Assessment and Counselling for Exercise and Nutrition (PACE) program Enhancement of physical activity and promotion of healthy nutrition habits	9 months	✓	✗	↓ % body fat and cholesterol	No specific dietary changes measured or reported

Note: Maintenance period refers to the time of evaluation in terms of the number of weeks or months after the intervention finished

Table 1. (Continued)

REFERENCE	POPULATION (Sample, Country, *N*, recruitment)	INTERVENTION	DURATION	POST-TEST	MAINTENANCE	RESULTS	COMMENTS
(Aldana, Greenlaw, Diehl, Englert, & Jackson, 2002)	Employees from various metropolitan companies U.S.A. 453 employees Voluntary participation	Coronary Health Improvement Project (CHIP) video program Health screen, recommendations from a nurse, 8 weeks of education delivered by video and facilitators Topics included dietary fibre, dietary fat, cholesterol, hypertension, diabetes education, & cancer	8 weeks	✓	✗	↓ BMI, weight, systolic and diastolic blood pressure, total cholesterol, HDL cholesterol, LDL cholesterol, triglycerides, and fasting blood glucose.	No control group
(Campbell et al., 2002)	Rural, female, blue-collar employees (manufacturing industries) U.S.A. 859 employees (660 at 6-months and 650 at 18 months)	Health Works for Women (HWW) Individualized computer-tailored health messages Natural helpers program (volunteers who enhance social support, promote activities, and share information) Physical activity, diet, smoking, breast and cervical cancer screening	18 months	✓	✗	1/3 way through (6 months from baseline): ↓ fat score Post-test: ↑ fruit & vegetables	

Note: Maintenance period refers to the time of evaluation in terms of the number of weeks or months after the intervention finished

Table 1. (Continued)

REFERENCE	POPULATION (Sample, Country, *N*, recruitment)	INTERVENTION	DURATION	POST-TEST	MAINTENANCE	RESULTS	COMMENTS
(Leslie, Lean, Baillie, & Hankey, 2002)	Male employees at a petrochemical worksite Scotland 122 employees (91 at post-test) Voluntary participation	Compared energy deficit diet with meat, energy deficit diet with no meat, low calorie diet with meat, and low calorie diet with no meat Dietary advice, eating plan	12 weeks	✓	✗	No differences between the groups Both groups combined: ↓ weight, BMI, waist, total cholesterol, LDL cholesterol, and triglycerides	
(Pegus, Bazzarre, Brown, & Menzin, 2002)	Employees from manufacturing worksites U.S.A. 663 employees Voluntary participation	Heart at Work program Exercise, low-fat diets, knowledge of risk factors	12 months	✓	✗	↑ knowledge of nutrition, diet, heart attack risk factors and blood pressure. More likely to report planning to change to a lower-fat diet or lose weight ↑ % reporting weight loss	

Note: Maintenance period refers to the time of evaluation in terms of the number of weeks or months after the intervention finished

Table 1. (Continued)

REFERENCE	POPULATION (Sample, Country, *N*, recruitment)	INTERVENTION	DURATION	POST-TEST	MAINTENANCE	RESULTS	COMMENTS
(Sorensen et al., 2002, 2003)	"Blue-collar workers" from manufacturing worksites U.S.A. 5156 employees (completing both baseline and post-test) Voluntary participation	WellWorks-2 study Health promotion or health promotion with integrated OH&S	2 years	✓	✗	No sig diff in fruit and vegetables	Comparing 2 intervention groups, no control group receiving a minimal intervention or no intervention at all
(Beresford et al., 2001)	Employees at worksites with cafeterias U.S.A. 1681 employees (completing both baseline and post-test)	Seattle 5 a Day Worksite Program Targeted to each worksite Individual behaviour change, and work environment Interventions for increasing fruit & veg consumption	2 years	✓	✗	↑ servings of fruit & vegetables	

Note: Maintenance period refers to the time of evaluation in terms of the number of weeks or months after the intervention finished

Table 1. (Continued)

REFERENCE	POPULATION (Sample, Country, *N*, recruitment)	INTERVENTION	DURATION	POST-TEST	MAINTENANCE	RESULTS	COMMENTS
(C. Cook, Simmons, Swinburn, & Stewart, 2001)	Male, hourly paid, employees at manufacturing worksites New Zealand 153 employees (136 after 6 month maintenance period) Voluntary participation	30 minute workshop session, once a month for 6 months Nutrition displays Heath promotion messages Water and low-fat items made available Nutrition, non-communicable disease risk, safe use of alcohol, and physical activity	6 months	✓	6 months (12 months from baseline)	↑ in vegetable servings, nutrition knowledge ↓ in systolic blood pressure, fat score No (significant) change in BMI, waist circumference, fruit servings, alcohol	
(Gordon et al., 2001)	Employees at companies in 3 cities U.S.A. 1483 employees	INTER$_x$VENT Cardiovascular disease risk reduction Risk appraisal, assessment, goal-setting, action plan implementation, long-term follow-up, compliance tracking Actions included referral to a dietician, nutrition and dietary supplements, physical activity etc.	12 weeks	✓	×	↓ total cholesterol, LDL cholesterol, triglycerides, and fasting blood glucose level	

Note: Maintenance period refers to the time of evaluation in terms of the number of weeks or months after the intervention finished

Table 1. (Continued)

REFERENCE	POPULATION (Sample, Country, *N*, recruitment)	INTERVENTION	DURATION	POST-TEST	MAINTENANCE	RESULTS	COMMENTS
(Parker et al., 2001)	U.S. Army War College U.S.A. (*N* not specified)	Interactive, educational training on: diet, stress management, cholesterol reduction, diabetes education, hypertension control, aerobic and strength training and others CD-ROM for nutrition education, health habits, aerobics and other areas Tailored program	not specified	not specified	not specified	No change in BMI Lower cholesterol than age-matched peers in the community Less than 2% of men and 4% of women exceed waist size recommendations	No control group Compared with rates in general population
(Pescatello et al., 2001)	Hospital employees U.S.A. 621 employees (278 over the 4 year intervention) Voluntary participation	Cardiovascular heart awareness program (CHAP) Cardiovascular screen, results counselling alone (CHAPonly) vs. cardiovascular screen, results counselling, structured health education and behavioural support program (CHAPplus)	4 years	✓	×	No significant differences between two groups of participants CHAP program led to improvements in blood glucose, LDL cholesterol and total cholesterol to HDL ratio	CHAPplus participants took part in exercise, nutrition and weight management, smoking cessation, OR cardiac rehabilitation. Some participants may not have participated in nutrition education

Note: Maintenance period refers to the time of evaluation in terms of the number of weeks or months after the intervention finished

Table 1. (Continued)

REFERENCE	POPULATION (Sample, Country, *N*, recruitment)	INTERVENTION	DURATION	POST-TEST	MAINTENANCE	RESULTS	COMMENTS
(Buller et al., 2000)	Public sector employees (e.g. government, public school, university employees) U.S.A. 331 employees (314 at 6 month maintenance period) completed evaluations	Arizona 5-a-day Peer Education Program Individuals who were central to social groups were trained as peer educators Peer educators engaged in nutrition education for 2 hours/week with co-workers Resource guide, newsletter, and enabling gifts (recipe book, seeds)	9 months	✓	6 months	Post-test: Contact with peer educators was associated with increases in fruit, vegetable and juice consumption Maintenance at 6 months: Contact with peer educators was associated with increases in fruit juice consumption	See Buller 1999 for direct impact on diet
(Holdsworth, Haslam, & Raymond, 2000)	Various workplaces England 1153 (577 at post-test) Voluntary participation	Heartbeat Award Scheme Reduction of coronary heart disease rates Nutrition goals: reduce fat, sugar and salt and increase fibre-rich, starchy foods	6 months	✓	×	↑ healthy eating information and availability of healthy foods at work No significant change in nutritional knowledge	

Note: Maintenance period refers to the time of evaluation in terms of the number of weeks or months after the intervention finished

Table 1. (Continued)

REFERENCE	POPULATION (Sample, Country, *N*, recruitment)	INTERVENTION	DURATION	POST-TEST	MAINTENANCE	RESULTS	COMMENTS
(Biener et al., 1999)	Employees from various worksites (manufacturing, communication, public service, and utilities) U.S.A. 20, 801 employees (18, 205 at follow-up after 3 years)	Working Well Trial Multi-site Targeted eating patterns at the individual level as well as changing the food environment (along with smoking and other risk factors)	not specified	not specified	(3 years from baseline)	↑ access to fruits and vegetables at work, ↑ access to nutrition information at work, ↑ nutrition labelling and changes in vending machines	
(Braeckman, De Bacquer, Maes, & De Backer, 1999)	Predominantly "blue-collar" male employees, aged 35-59, from Belgian worksites Belgium 770 employees (638 at post-test) Voluntary participation	Nutrition education program Health screening, individual counselling and feedback Information, posters, video, 2 hour education session and a newsletter Targets: lowering fat and cholesterol	3 months	✓	✗	↑ nutrition knowledge ↑ proteins and carbohydrates ↓ total calories and % of energy from fat Only ↓ cholesterol in those with hypercholesterolemia	

Note: Maintenance period refers to the time of evaluation in terms of the number of weeks or months after the intervention finished

Table 1. (Continued)

REFERENCE	POPULATION (Sample, Country, *N*, recruitment)	INTERVENTION	DURATION	POST-TEST	MAINTENANCE	RESULTS	COMMENTS
(Brug, 1999)	Employees of an oil company, a health care organisation and healthy volunteers (results from three studies combined) The Netherlands 1309 participants	Computer-tailored nutrition advice) vs. tailored feedback letters vs. general non-tailored feedback letters	not specified	✓	✗	Computer-tailored advice: ↓ fat scores from pre to post assessments (not significantly different from other groups) Tailored advice (computer or letter): more likely to read and discuss the nutrition advice	Employees and community sample

Note: Maintenance period refers to the time of evaluation in terms of the number of weeks or months after the intervention finished

Table 1. (Continued)

REFERENCE	POPULATION (Sample, Country, *N*, recruitment)	INTERVENTION	DURATION	POST-TEST	MAINTENANCE	RESULTS	COMMENTS
(Buller et al., 1999)	Employees from a multicultural, lower-income population U.S.A. 2091 employees (695 at post-test) Note: 1523 employees not randomized because not in a "clique" eligible for peer education Voluntary participation	Five a Day Education Program with a peer health education program vs. Five a Day Education Program alone Workplace mail, cafeteria promotions, and speakers Peer educators identified using social network analysis Peer educator training Informal conversations with peers about eating fruits and vegetables	18 months	✓	6 months	Post-test: ↑ fruits and vegetables ↑ awareness of the 5 a Day program, knowledge of appropriate number of servings of fruit and veg Improved diet-related attitudes Maintenance at 6 months: Total number of servings, awareness of the 5 a Day program, knowledge of appropriate number of servings of fruit and veg per day persisted Some diet-related attitudes Perception that fruits and vegetables = easy to get at work	

Note: Maintenance period refers to the time of evaluation in terms of the number of weeks or months after the intervention finished

Table 1. (Continued)

REFERENCE	POPULATION (Sample, Country, *N*, recruitment)	INTERVENTION	DURATION	POST-TEST	MAINTENANCE	RESULTS	COMMENTS
(Emmons, Linnan, Shadel, Marcus, & Abrams, 1999)	University School of medicine/hospital employees U.S.A. 2291 employees	Working health project/working well trial Workers participated in design and implementation Nutrition, smoking and physical activity Nutrition focused on fat, fibre, fruits and vegetables	2.5 years	✓	✗	small ↑ fruit and veg ↑ fibre No differences in fat intake between the intervention and control groups	
(Fries, Ripley, Figueiredo, & Thompson, 1999)	Employees of rural manufacturing companies U.S.A. 217 employees (184 employees at post-test) Voluntary participation (although some information distributed to all employees)	Intervention on smoking and diet Posters, dietary information, cancer prevention library, computerised dietary fat screening with personalised dietary feedback, nutrition seminar	9 months	✓	✗	↑ reported likelihood of reducing dietary fat and confidence of doing so ↑ servings of fruit and vegetables ↑ perceived support at work for reducing fat intake	No control group

Note: Maintenance period refers to the time of evaluation in terms of the number of weeks or months after the intervention finished

Table 1. (Continued)

REFERENCE	POPULATION (Sample, Country, *N*, recruitment)	INTERVENTION	DURATION	POST-TEST	MAINTENANCE	RESULTS	COMMENTS
(Sorensen et al., 1999)	Employees from health centres U.S.A. 1359 employees (1306 at 1-2 month maintenance period)	Treatwell 5-a-day study Minimal intervention vs. worksite vs. worksite with family involvement 5-a-day media campaign, promotion of the Cancer Information Service Hotline, 1 hour nutrition presentation and taste test at the worksite Work: Individual behaviour change and changes in the worksite environment Family: “learn at home program”, annual family newsletter, annual family festival, materials mailed to families	19.5 months	✖ (see maintenance)	1-2 months (22 months post-baseline)	↑ fruit and veg in intervention groups after controlling for gender, education, occupation, race/ethnicity, and living situation Change was largest in work + family support intervention.	

Note: Maintenance period refers to the time of evaluation in terms of the number of weeks or months after the intervention finished

Table 1. (Continued)

REFERENCE	POPULATION (Sample, Country, *N*, recruitment)	INTERVENTION	DURATION	POST-TEST	MAINTENANCE	RESULTS	COMMENTS
(Talvi, Jarvisalo, & Knuts, 1999)	Employees of two oil refineries Finland 885 employees (798 at 3 years) Voluntary participation	Group A: counselling Group B: feedback and instructions given in written format For those with goals relating to diet there was a lecture covering energy intake and consumption, BMI, metabolism and healthy cooking Physical activity, dietary habits, obesity, blood pressure, serum lipids and smoking Health examination Health goals	3 years	✓	×	↓ BMI in men in both groups and ↑ BMI in women in group B ↓ HDL-cholesterol in men in both groups and women in group B ↓ serum cholesterol in men in group B	

Note: Maintenance period refers to the time of evaluation in terms of the number of weeks or months after the intervention finished

Other studies achieved differences in BMI but did not include a maintenance period in their research design (Aldana et al., 2002; Leslie et al., 2002). Talvi et al. (1999) found a reduction in BMI but only in men for two interventions: counselling, and written feedback and instructions based on a health examination. Petersen et al. (2008) also found a reduction in weight as a result of an online weight management program that persisted during a 6 month maintenance period. However, this study did not use a control group. An evaluation of the program after a 12 month maintenance period with a control group did not find a significant difference in the weight of those who participated in the program.

Problems Experienced in Delivering Workplace Programs

Retention

Retaining participants in nutrition education or health promotion programs was a challenge for several programs. Despite the importance of this issue, many studies did not report retention rates in their papers. Where they were reported, levels of drop-outs were sometimes high. For example, Holdsworth et al. (2000) and Block et al. (2004) reported that only 50% and 56% of participants completed all stages of their respective programs, including all of the evaluations. On the basis of these participation rates, it is important to observe that even if these nutrition education programs significantly improve the health and wellbeing of some employees, these effects may not generalize to the whole workforce. Participation in nutrition education sessions is often on a voluntary basis and as such, caters for people who are already interested in nutrition and/or motivated to change their health behaviour. Thus, these interventions do not reach people who are less motivated and who may stand the most to gain from nutrition education. The specific reasons for low retention rates should be determined in order to make nutrition education interesting and relevant to a larger number of people. In addition, it is important to remember that the results from program evaluations may be amplified if they only include those who like the program and therefore, complete the program, in the assessment of the program's outcomes.

Program Duration and Long-Term Change

The majority of the nutrition education or health promotion programs were evaluated at their conclusion without any further follow-up (Abood et al., 2003; Aldana et al., 2002; Atlantis et al., 2006; Beresford et al., 2001; Block et al., 2004; Block et al., 2008; Braeckman et al., 1999; Brug, 1999; Campbell et al., 2002; Chen et al., 2008; R. F. Cook et al., 2007; Cousineau et al., 2008; Elliot et al., 2004; Emmons et al., 1999; Engbers et al., 2006; Fries et al., 1999; Gill & Wijk, 2004; Gordon et al., 2001; Holdsworth et al., 2000; Holdsworth et al., 2004; Leslie et al., 2002; Moy et al., 2006; Pegus et al., 2002; Pescatello et al., 2001; Polacsek et al., 2006; Proper et al., 2003; Renaud et al., 2008; Shimizu et al., 2004; Sorensen et al., 2002; Sorensen et al., 2003; Sorensen et al., 2005; Sorensen et al., 2007; Steenhuis et al., 2004; Talvi et al., 1999; Williams et al., 2004; Yancey et al., 2006). As a result, the extent to which dietary changes were maintained over time is unknown. Furthermore, several studies did not explicitly state the duration of their interventions, making it unclear whether the evaluations were conducted during the intervention period, at its conclusion, or at a later follow-up (Biener et al., 1999; De Bourdeaudhuij et al., 2007; Parker et al., 2001; Williams et al., 2004).

Despite these limitations, a few studies evaluated the programs 6 months after their completion (Aldana et al., 2005; Buller et al., 2000; Buller et al., 1999; C. Cook et al., 2001; Muto & Yamauchi, 2001; Sorensen et al., 1999). In general, these studies had encouraging results with increased fruit and vegetable consumption (Aldana et al., 2005; Buller et al., 2000; Buller et al., 1999; C. Cook et al., 2001; Sorensen et al., 1999), decreased fat and red meat intake (Aldana et al., 2005), reduced blood pressure (C. Cook et al., 2001), and cholesterol (Aldana et al., 2005). Buller et al. (1999) found that while some effects persisted after 6 months (awareness of the program, knowledge of the appropriate number of daily servings of fruit and vegetables) others did not, such as increased consumption of fruit and vegetables. This study indicates that behavioural change may be more difficult to maintain over time than changes in knowledge and awareness.

In addition, there were conflicting results regarding BMI. Although Cook et al. (2001) found no difference in BMI or waist circumference, some of the studies with a pre-test post-test design without long term follow-up, found significant reductions in BMI (Aldana et al., 2002; Leslie et al., 2002). Furthermore, Aldana et al. (2005) found reduced BMI after a 5 month maintenance period. In contrast, one study (Prior et al., 2005) had a follow-up period of over three years and found reduced diastolic blood pressure but found increases in BMI and weight in men and women, and an increase in cholesterol in women. Although this is discouraging in terms of long term change this intervention was very brief. It is not clear whether inconsistent results with respect to BMI are due to differences in the programs that were implemented or differences in the program participants.

In sum, there is limited evidence of long term change as a result of nutrition education and health promotion programs in the workplace. However, this may result from the study designs that have been utilised and the small number of studies with extensive longitudinal follow-up. Future studies should endeavour to follow-up participants over a period of months, and possibly years, because nutrition education aims to improve or change eating habits in the long-term. Nutrition education programs may need to consider additional sessions, updates or different approaches for keeping employees motivated, to maintain the changes that are achieved over a longer period of time.

Study Design

The benefits of nutrition education programs can be difficult to determine due to the manner in which they are evaluated. Many of the studies included in the current review did not include a control group and therefore would not meet minimal requirements for evaluation of program efficacy. Without a control group it is not possible to determine whether changes in dietary habits have resulted from factors such as the participants' awareness that they were being studied, health promotion efforts in the community such as media campaigns, or seasonal changes, such as increased caloric intake in autumn and decreased intake in spring (Ma et al., 2006). A control group would account for these possibilities because control participants would also have been aware of their involvement in research, they would have been exposed to other health promotion efforts, and may have participated at the same time of year as those in a nutrition education program. The inclusion of a control group is therefore a basic requirement for good internal validity and, consequently, demonstration of program efficacy.

In addition, some studies relied primarily on self-report measures of diet, while others included health outcomes, which should reflect dietary behaviour, such as cholesterol and BMI. A reliance on the former alone, as the main outcome of the interventions raises the possibility of "social desirability bias" confounding the outcome (Fisher, 1993). Participants may want to make a good impression by being seen to do the "right" thing (e.g. eat more fruits and vegetables) and not to do the "wrong" thing (e.g. consume foods that are high in fat) and respond accordingly on self-report measures. Furthermore, health outcomes may not reflect dietary changes accurately because changes in BMI and cholesterol may not be seen straight away and other aspects of health may affect these outcomes such as thyroid disorders and diabetes. Ideally, both forms of measurement should be included. Despite their limitations, if self-report measures and health measures yield consistent results, the intervention is more likely to have resulted in significant change.

Multiple Health Behaviours

Nutrition education was not necessarily the primary focus of the health promotion programs that were evaluated by the studies included in this review, although it was an important component of these programs. The majority of the interventions targeted more than one health behaviour such as diet, physical activity, and smoking. There is growing evidence that interventions that target multiple health behaviours are equally or more effective than those that target single health behaviours (for a review refer to Prochaska, Spring, & Nigg, 2008). This may be because unhealthy behaviours often co-occur. That is, people who have an unhealthy diet may also be physically inactive and smoke. Similarly, achieving change in one area of health may lead to increased confidence in one's ability to improve behaviour in another (Prochaska et al., 2008). Therefore, change to unhealthy behaviours may also co-occur. Interventions that focus on multiple health behaviours also make sense on a practical level due to the expense and time involved in health promotion.

New Areas of Investigation

Studies described in this review have tended to focus on a limited number of mechanisms for achieving behaviour change; education delivered through a variety of methods (information sheets, telephone, computer, face-to-face etc), individual feedback and goal setting, counselling, and use of peer educators and social support.

Only a few studies looked to employer-initiated, fundamental changes to the worksite as a way to ameliorate environmental barriers to behaviour change. These sorts of initiatives have been defined by Glanz et al. (1996) as those strategies that do not require individuals to self-select into defined educational programs. Examples of such initiatives tend to generally focus on top-down alterations to the entire workplace environment. They include studies in which healthy foods are made more accessible and information about their value is provided

(Biener et al., 1999; Dawson, Dwyer, Evers, & Sheeshka, 2006; Engbers et al., 2006; Gill & Wijk, 2004; Steenhuis et al., 2004). These approaches go some way towards addressing the recommendations of the International Labour Organisation (ILO) who, in 1956 promulgated the Welfare Facilities Recommendation (No. 102), in which guidelines for the establishments of workplace canteens were provided. Although the original focus of the ILO was on malnutrition, in the current context, workplace practices that address over-nutrition could assist in alleviating concerns with employee overweight. A recent expert report on cancer prevention from the World Cancer Research Fund (2009) recommends that workplaces encourage healthy eating habits by using incentives, removal of foods that are high in salt, sugar, or fat from vending machines, provision of healthy food options in cafeterias, and provision of nutrition education and information on disease prevention.

Some workplaces are already firmly committed to the establishment of an organisational climate that supports "healthy weight". For example, a number of autoworker unions have successfully lobbied for employer supported food programs for their workers, with the Canadian Auto Workers achieving a "better meals" program for employees of Chrysler in 2001 and General Motors in 2004 (Wanjek, 2005). In Denmark, a small, employer-sponsored intervention in which free fruit was supplied to employees in 6 worksites and subsequent intake was compared between these and 6 control settings, proved so successful that by 2004, 9288 worksites were participating in like programs representing 9% of workplaces in Denmark (http://6omdagen.dk/foredrag/2005VIEsymposiumMM3.ppt).

Future studies might usefully further compare worksites where the environmental context is altered so that workplace practices support healthy dietary choices to the more traditional workplace setting. The precise nature of these changes might vary but they are likely to include employer subsidization of healthy food choices including, but not limited to, the removal of the sale of snack foods, provision of fruit and bottled water free of charge, and labelling of healthy food items.

CONCLUSIONS

Nutrition education is a central component to many health promotion programs that take place in the workplace. The workplace is a useful setting for providing information and support for healthy behaviours because many people spend a large amount of their time at work and it provides a context that can provide supportive social norms.

Although this review was limited to published studies, which may be biased towards studies with significant findings, the available evidence suggests that nutrition education in the workplace is successful in achieving improvements in diet. However, more longitudinal studies are necessary to support a reliable assessment of whether these programs achieve enduring weight loss. Limited evidence indicates that interventions that utilise web-based approaches hold promise due to their accessibility and affordability. In addition, peer-based approaches, which take advantage of existing social networks, may appeal as an alternative to programs that appear driven by management. This review indicates that although nutrition education in the workplace leads to promising outcomes, further research is necessary to address issues of participant retention and long-term maintenance of changes to dietary habits.

The effectiveness of workplace based environmental interventions must be subjected to the same scrutiny of design, sample and effectiveness as that applied to small, one-off programs. However, it is also important to realise that translational research requires high level ecological validation as well as internal validation, and the two may conflict. In other words, a well-controlled study where confounds are minimised, where dependent and independent measures are well-defined and measured, and where treatments are not contaminated, may produce a significant effect, but it may be impossible to initiate this treatment in the "real-world" environment or to maintain it through time or across work settings and employee groups.

References

Abood, D. A., Black, D. R., & Feral, D. (2003). Nutrition education worksite intervention for university staff: application of the health belief model. *J Nutr Educ Behav, 35(5),* 260-267.

Aldana, S. G., Greenlaw, R., Diehl, H. A., Englert, H., & Jackson, R. (2002). Impact of the coronary health improvement project (CHIP) on several employee populations. *J Occup Environ Med, 44(9),* 831-839.

Aldana, S. G., Greenlaw, R. L., Diehl, H. A., Salberg, A., Merrill, R. M., & Ohmine, S. (2005). The effects of a worksite chronic disease prevention program. *J Occup Environ Med, 47(6),* 558-564.

Atlantis, E., Chow, C. M., Kirby, A., & Fiatarone Singh, M. A. (2006). Worksite intervention effects on physical health: a randomized controlled trial. *Health Promot Int, 21(3),* 191-200.

Beresford, S. A., Thompson, B., Feng, Z., Christianson, A., McLerran, D., & Patrick, D. L. (2001). Seattle 5 a Day worksite program to increase fruit and vegetable consumption. *Prev Med, 32(3),* 230-238.

Biener, L., Glanz, K., McLerran, D., Sorensen, G., Thompson, B., Basen-Engquist, K., et al. (1999). Impact of the Working Well Trial on the worksite smoking and nutrition environment. *Health Educ Behav, 26(4),* 478-494.

Block, G., Block, T., Wakimoto, P., & Block, C. H. (2004). Demonstration of an E-mailed worksite nutrition intervention program. *Prev Chronic Dis, 1(4),* A06.

Block, G., Sternfeld, B., Block, C. H., Block, T. J., Norris, J., Hopkins, D., et al. (2008). Development of Alive! (A Lifestyle Intervention Via Email), and its effect on health-related quality of life, presenteeism, and other behavioral outcomes: randomized controlled trial. *J Med Internet Res, 10,(4),* e43.

Braeckman, L., De Bacquer, D., Maes, L., & De Backer, G. (1999). Effects of a low-intensity worksite-based nutrition intervention. *Occup Med (Lond), 49(8),* 549-555.

Brug, J. (1999). Dutch research into the development and impact of computer-tailored nutrition education. *Eur J Clin Nutr, 53 Suppl 2,* S78-82.

Buller, D., Buller, M. K., Larkey, L., Sennott-Miller, L., Taren, D., Aickin, M., et al. (2000). Implementing a 5-a-day peer health educator program for public sector labor and trades employees. *Health Educ Behav, 27(2),* 232-240.

Buller, D., Morrill, C., Taren, D., Aickin, M., Sennott-Miller, L., Buller, M. K., et al. (1999). Randomized trial testing the effect of peer education at increasing fruit and vegetable intake. *J Natl Cancer Inst, 91(17),* 1491-1500.

Campbell, M. K., Tessaro, I., DeVellis, B., Benedict, S., Kelsey, K., Belton, L., et al. (2002). Effects of a tailored health promotion program for female blue-collar workers: health works for women. *Prev Med, 34(3),* 313-323.

Chen, J., Wu, X., & Gu, D. (2008). Hypertension and cardiovascular diseases intervention in the capital steel and iron company and Beijing Fangshan community. *Obes Rev, 9 Suppl 1,* 142-145.

Cook, C., Simmons, G., Swinburn, B., & Stewart, J. (2001). Changing risk behaviours for non-communicable disease in New Zealand working men--is workplace intervention effective? *N Z Med J, 114(1130),* 175-178.

Cook, R. F., Billings, D. W., Hersch, R. K., Back, A. S., & Hendrickson, A. (2007). A field test of a web-based workplace health promotion program to improve dietary practices, reduce stress, and increase physical activity: randomized controlled trial. *J Med Internet Res, 9(2),* e17.

Cousineau, T., Houle, B., Bromberg, J., Fernandez, K. C. & Kling, W. C. (2008). A pilot study of an online workplace nutrition program: the value of participant input in program development. *J Nutr Educ Behav, 40(3),* 160-167.

Dalziel, K. & Segal, L. (2007). Time to give nutrition interventions a higher profile: cost-effectiveness of 10 nutrition interventions. *Health Promot Int, 22(4),* 271-283.

Dawson, J., Dwyer, J. J., Evers, S. & Sheeshka, J. (2006). Eat smart! Workplace Cafeteria Program evaluation of the nutrition component. *Can J Diet Pract Res, 67(2),* 85-90.

De Bourdeaudhuij, I., Stevens, V., Vandelanotte, C. & Brug, J. (2007). Evaluation of an interactive computer-tailored nutrition intervention in a real-life setting. *Ann Behav Med, 33(1),* 39-48.

Elliot, D. L., Goldberg, L., Duncan, T. E., Kuehl, K. S., Moe, E. L., Breger, R. K., et al. (2004). The PHLAME firefighters' study: feasibility and findings. *Am J Health Behav, 28*(1), 13-23.

Emmons, K. M., Linnan, L. A., Shadel, W. G., Marcus, B. & Abrams, D. B. (1999). The Working Healthy Project: a worksite health-promotion trial targeting physical activity, diet, and smoking. *J Occup Environ Med, 41(7),* 545-555.

Engbers, L. H., Van Poppel, M. N., Chin, A. P. M. & Van Mechelen, W. (2006). The effects of a controlled worksite environmental intervention on determinants of dietary behavior and self-reported fruit, vegetable and fat intake. *BMC Public Health, 6*, 253.

Fisher, R. J. (1993). Social desirability bias and the validity of indirect questioning. *Journal of Consumer Research, 20*, 303-315.

Fries, E. A., Ripley, J. S., Figueiredo, M. I. & Thompson, B. (1999). Can community organization strategies be used to implement smoking and dietary changes in a rural manufacturing work site? *J Rural Health, 15(4),* 413-420.

Gill, P. E. & Wijk, K. (2004). Case study of a healthy eating intervention for Swedish lorry drivers. *Health Educ Res, 19(3),* 306-315.

Glanz, K., Sorensen, G. & Farmer, A. (1996). The health impact of worksite nutrition and cholesterol intervention programs. *Am J Health Promot, 10(6),* 453-470.

Gordon, N. F., Salmon, R. D., Mitchell, B. S., Faircloth, G. C., Levinrad, L. I., Salmon, S., et al. (2001). Innovative approaches to comprehensive cardiovascular disease risk reduction in clinical and community-based settings. *Curr Atheroscler Rep, 3(6),* 498-506.

Holdsworth, M., Haslam, C. & Raymond, N. T. (2000). Does the heartbeat award scheme change employees' dietary attitudes and knowledge? *Appetite, 35(2),* 179-188.

Holdsworth, M., Raymond, N. T. & Haslam, C. (2004). Does the Heartbeat Award scheme in England result in change in dietary behaviour in the workplace? *Health Promot Int, 19(2),* 197-204.

Kumanyika, S. K., Obarzanek, E., Stettler, N., Bell, R., Field, A. E., Fortmann, S. P., et al. (2008). Population-based prevention of obesity: the need for comprehensive promotion of healthful eating, physical activity, and energy balance: a scientific statement from American Heart Association Council on Epidemiology and Prevention, Interdisciplinary Committee for Prevention (formerly the expert panel on population and prevention science). *Circulation, 118(4),* 428-464.

Leslie, W. S., Lean, M. E., Baillie, H. M. & Hankey, C. R. (2002). Weight management: a comparison of existing dietary approaches in a work-site setting. *Int J Obes Relat Metab Disord, 26(11),* 1469-1475.

Ma, Y., Olendzki, B. C., Li, W., Hafner, A. R., Chiriboga, D., Hebert, J. R., et al. (2006). Seasonal variation in food intake, physical activity, and body weight in a predominantly overweight population. *Eur J Clin Nutr, 60(4),* 519-528.

McMillan, D. C., Sattar, N. & McArdle, C. S. (2006). ABC of obesity. Obesity and cancer. *Bmj, 333*(7578), 1109-1111.

Moy, F., Sallam, A. A. & Wong, M. (2006). The results of a worksite health promotion programme in Kuala Lumpur, Malaysia. *Health Promot Int, 21(4),* 301-310.

Must, A., Spadano, J., Coakley, E. H., Field, A. E., Colditz, G. & Dietz, W. H. (1999). The disease burden associated with overweight and obesity. *Jama, 282(16),* 1523-1529.

Muto, T., & Yamauchi, K. (2001). Evaluation of a multicomponent workplace health promotion program conducted in Japan for improving employees' cardiovascular disease risk factors. *Prev Med, 33(6),* 571-577.

National Audit Office. (2004). Obesity. Third report of session 2003-2004. The House of Commons Health Committee. [Electronic Version]. Retrieved 29th January 2009 from http://www.publications.parliament.uk/pa/cm200304/cmselect/cmhealth/23/23.pdf.

Papadaki, A. & Scott, J. A. (2008). Follow-up of a web-based tailored intervention promoting the Mediterranean diet in Scotland. *Patient Educ Couns.*

Parker, M. W., Fuller, G. F., Koenig, H. G., Bellis, J. M., Vaitkus, M. A., Barko, W. F., et al. (2001). Soldier and family wellness across the life course: a developmental model of successful aging, spirituality, and health promotion, Part II. *Mil Med, 166(7),* 561-570.

Pegus, C., Bazzarre, T. L., Brown, J. S. & Menzin, J. (2002). Effect of the Heart At Work program on awareness of risk factors, self-efficacy, and health behaviors. *J Occup Environ Med, 44(3),* 228-236.

Pescatello, L. S., Murphy, D., Vollono, J., Lynch, E., Bernene, J. & Costanzo, D. (2001). The cardiovascular health impact of an incentive worksite health promotion program. *Am J Health Promot, 16(1),* 16-20.

Petersen, R., Sill, S., Lu, C., Young, J. & Edington, D. W. (2008). Effectiveness of employee internet-based weight management program. *J Occup Environ Med, 50(2),* 163-171.

Plotnikoff, R. C., McCargar, L. J., Wilson, P. M. & Loucaides, C. A. (2005). Efficacy of an E-mail intervention for the promotion of physical activity and nutrition behavior in the workplace context. *Am J Health Promot, 19(6),* 422-429.

Polacsek, M., O'Brien, L. M., Lagasse, W. & Hammar, N. (2006). Move & Improve: a worksite wellness program in Maine. *Prev Chronic Dis, 3(3),* A101.

Prior, J. O., van Melle, G., Crisinel, A., Burnand, B., Cornuz, J. & Darioli, R. (2005). Evaluation of a multicomponent worksite health promotion program for cardiovascular risk factors-correcting for the regression towards the mean effect. *Prev Med, 40(3),* 259-267.

Prochaska, J. J., Spring, B. & Nigg, C. R. (2008). Multiple health behavior change research: an introduction and overview. *Prev Med, 46(3),* 181-188.

Proper, K. I., Hildebrandt, V. H., Van der Beek, A. J., Twisk, J. W. & Van Mechelen, W. (2003). Effect of individual counseling on physical activity fitness and health: a randomized controlled trial in a workplace setting. *Am J Prev Med, 24(3),* 218-226.

Renaud, L., Kishchuk, N., Juneau, M., Nigam, A., Tereault, K. & Leblanc, M. C. (2008). Implementation and outcomes of a comprehensive worksite health promotion program. *Can J Public Health, 99(1),* 73-77.

Rosenthal, R. (1995). Writing meta-analytic reviews. *Psychologcial Bulletin, 118(2),* 183-192.

Shimizu, T., Horiguchi, I., Kato, T. & Nagata, S. (2004). Relationship between an interview-based health promotion program and cardiovascular risk factors at Japanese companies. *J Occup Health, 46(3),* 205-212.

Sorensen, G., Barbeau, E., Stoddard, A. M., Hunt, M. K., Kaphingst, K. & Wallace, L. (2005). Promoting behavior change among working-class, multiethnic workers: results of the healthy directions--small business study. *Am J Public Health, 95(8),* 1389-1395.

Sorensen, G., Stoddard, A., Peterson, K., Cohen, N., Hunt, M. K., Stein, E., et al. (1999). Increasing fruit and vegetable consumption through worksites and families in the treatwell 5-a-day study. *Am J Public Health, 89*(1), 54-60.

Sorensen, G., Stoddard, A. M., Dubowitz, T., Barbeau, E. M., Bigby, J., Emmons, K. M., et al. (2007). The influence of social context on changes in fruit and vegetable consumption: results of the healthy directions studies. *Am J Public Health, 97(7),* 1216-1227.

Sorensen, G., Stoddard, A. M., LaMontagne, A. D., Emmons, K., Hunt, M. K., Youngstrom, R., et al. (2002). A comprehensive worksite cancer prevention intervention: behavior change results from a randomized controlled trial (United States). *Cancer Causes Control, 13(6),* 493-502.

Sorensen, G., Stoddard, A. M., LaMontagne, A. D., Emmons, K., Hunt, M. K., Youngstrom, R., et al. (2003). A comprehensive worksite cancer prevention intervention: behavior change results from a randomized controlled trial (United States). *J Public Health Policy, 24(1),* 5-25.

Spraycar, M. (Ed). (1995). *Stedman's Medical Dictionary.* 26th edn. Baltimore: Williams & Wilkins.

Steenhuis, I., Van Assema, P., Van Breukelen, G., Glanz, K., Kok, G. & De Vries, H. (2004). The impact of educational and environmental interventions in Dutch worksite cafeterias. *Health Promot Int, 19(3),* 335-343.

Talvi, A. I., Jarvisalo, J. O. & Knuts, L. R. (1999). A health promotion programme for oil refinery employees: changes of health promotion needs observed at three years. *Occup Med (Lond), 49(2),* 93-101.

Wanjek, C. (2005). Food at work: Workplace Solutions for Malnutrition, Obesity and Chronic Diseases. International Labour Office.

Williams, A., Wold, J., Dunkin, J., Idleman, L. & Jackson, C. (2004). CVD prevention strategies with urban and rural African American women. *Appl Nurs Res, 17(3),* 187-194.

World Cancer Research Fund / American Institute for Cancer Research (2009). Policy and Action for Cancer Prevention. Food, Nutrition, and Physical Activity: a Global Perspective. Washington DC: AICR.

Yancey, A. K., Lewis, L. B., Guinyard, J. J., Sloane, D. C., Nascimento, L. M., Galloway-Gilliam, L., et al. (2006). Putting promotion into practice: the African Americans building a legacy of health organizational wellness program. *Health Promot Pract, 7*(3 Suppl), 233S-246S.

In: Nutritional Education
Editor: Ida R. Laidyth

ISBN: 978-1-60876-078-7

Chapter 3

NUTRITION EDUCATION IN SCHOOL-BASED CHILDHOOD AND ADOLESCENT OBESITY PREVENTION PROGRAMS

Melinda J. Ickes[1] and Manoj Sharma[2]

[1]Graduate Assistant, Health Promotion & Education, University of Cincinnati, PO Box 210068, Cincinnati, OH 45221-0068, USA

[2]Professor, Health Promotion & Education, University of Cincinnati, PO Box 210068 Cincinnati, OH 45221-0068, USA

ABSTRACT

The purpose of this chapter was to review nutrition education in school-based childhood and adolescent obesity prevention programs. Problems of overweight and obesity have reached epidemic proportions in children and adolescents. With the large number of children and adolescents affected by overweight and obesity, it has been recognized as a critical public health threat, and prevention should become a priority. Schools have been considered an important venue for the delivery of health education programs since a majority of the nation's youth can be reached. Implementing a program in the school does not necessarily correspond to success, and therefore common components among successful nutrition education programs were examined. Providing age-appropriate, culturally sensitive instruction and materials were connected to the success of the programs. Success was also found when the nutrition education program was relevant to the student, and information was applicable to their everyday life. It was also critical to go beyond dissemination of knowledge and develop attitudes, skills, and behaviors to adopt, maintain, and enjoy healthy nutrition habits. Finally, recommendations were made to enhance the effectiveness of future school-based nutrition education programs.

Corresponding Author: [1](859) 572-5196 (Phone),(513) 556-3898 (Fax), ickesmj@uc.edu (e-mail)
[2](513) 556-3878 (Phone), (513) 556-3898 (Fax), manoj.sharma@uc.edu (e-mail)

Introduction

Prevalence

Problems of overweight and obesity have reached epidemic proportions (Ogden, Flegal, Carroll, & Johnson, 2002). Globally, approximately 1.6 billion adults (age 15+) were classified as overweight and of those at least 400 million were obese (World Health Organization, 2005). The World Health Organization projects these statistics to increase; by 2015, approximately 2.3 billion adults will be overweight and more than 700 million will be obese all over the world. In the United States, obesity prevalence doubled among adults between 1980 and 2004. More than one-third of adults, or over 72 million people, were obese in 2005-2006, including 33.3% among adult men and 33.2% among adult women (U.S. Department of Health and Human Services, 2007).

Unfortunately, the obesity epidemic has not been limited to adults but the percentage of children and adolescents who were overweight has also continued to increase. Obesity has been one of the most widespread health threats facing children and adolescents (Evans, Finkelstein, Kamerow & Renaud, 2005). Many health professionals have considered it to be a serious health issue which has placed a burden on our society. In the United States, childhood obesity was defined as being at or above the 95th percentile according to the Centers for Disease Control and Prevention (CDC) age-and gender-specific body mass index charts. Those considered at-risk for overweight were at or above the 85th percentile and below the 95th percentile (CDC, 2005).

According to the 2005-2006 National Health and Nutrition Examination Survey (NHANES) data, among 2-19 year old children, 17.1% were considered overweight: 13.9% of 2-5 year old, 18.8% of 6-11 year old, and 17.4% of 12-19 year old children (CDC, 2005). Variances exist among the states, with seven states incurring obesity rates of 15% - 19%. Among children and teenagers aged 6 - 19, 16% (almost 9 million) were overweight (CDC, 2005; Kaufman, 2003; USDHHS, 2004, 2007). This suggested that overall, 10% of the school-aged children in the world were overweight (Lobstein, Baur, Uauy, & IASO International Obesity Task Force, 2004). There has been a strong link between obesity during childhood and adolescence into adulthood, making the prevention of obesity in these populations a priority (Wilson, 2008).

Consequences of Child and Adolescent Obesity

Child and adolescent obesity has been of concern to many health professionals, parents, teachers, and school administrators because of the negative impact on the child's physical, psychological, behavioral, and social health. See Table 1 for a summary of these consequences. Children who were overweight had five times the risk of low health-related quality of life compared to children of normal weight (Schwimmer, Burwinkle, & Varni, 2003).

Physical Consequences. The dangers of being overweight or obese in childhood and adolescence have been well established. The Bogalusa Heart Study conducted in the United

States found that by 10 years of age, 60% of overweight children had at least one biochemical or clinical cardiovascular risk factor and 25% had more than two (Freedman, Dietz, Srinivasan, & Berenson, 1999). Additional long-term health consequences of childhood overweight included an increased risk of developing high blood pressure, high cholesterol, type 2 diabetes, stroke, certain types of cancer, gallbladder disease, arthritis, sleep disturbances, and asthma (USDHHS, 2007). Reportedly, physicians were increasingly treating pediatric patients who displayed symptoms of chronic diseases previously associated primarily with adulthood. Children were displaying conditions associated with serious health threats and a decreased life span (Shelton, 2008).

In addition, those who were overweight during childhood were more likely to maintain obesity into adulthood (Whitaker, Wright, Pepe, Seidel, & Dietz, 1997). In fact, a comprehensive review of the literature on childhood overweight persisting into adulthood indicated that 42% - 63% of overweight school-age children became obese adults, and the risk of obesity in adulthood was at least twice as high for overweight children as for non-overweight children (Smith, 2004). For the first time in history, the steady increase in life expectancy was threatened by a generation who would more than likely live unhealthier and shorter lives than their parents (Wilson, 2008).

Psychological Consequences. Children and adolescents who were overweight also experienced a variety of psychosocial issues: depression, peer rejection, low self-esteem, stigmatization, and discrimination (Erickson, Robinson, Haydel, & Killen, 2000; Schwartz & Puhl, 2003; Strauss, 2000). A widespread stereotype and negative attitude towards overweight and obese individuals has led to discrimination, as well as feelings of shame and guilt amongst these individuals (Cossrow, Jeffrey, & McGuire, 2001). Only a few studies have been reported on the topic of overweight stigmatization, but common threads of prejudicial treatment and discrimination were apparent. This stigmatization led to the internalization of negative self-evaluations which typically resulted in self-rejection. According to Charles Horton Cooley's (1964) looking-glass self theory, we see ourselves as others see us. Thus, children dealing with weight issues were exposed to a negative environment, which tended to be detrimental to their psychological and social functioning.

Societal Consequences. The effects of obesity on society were also indicated, primarily by imposing a significant financial burden on the health-care system. In the United States, the national health care expenditures related to overweight and obesity in adults were estimated between $98 billion and $129 billion (Institute of Medicine, 2004). Over the past two decades, costs associated with obesity-related illnesses specifically in children rose from $35 million to $127 million. States' annual medical spending for prevention, diagnosis, and treatment of individuals with obesity was estimated to range from $87 million to $7.7 billion across various states (Pyle, Sharkey, Yetter, Felix, & Furlong, 2006). Medical costs associated with overweight and obesity involved both direct and indirect costs. According to Finkelstein, Fiebelkorn and Wang (2003), direct medical costs included preventive, diagnostic, and treatment services. In contrast, indirect costs were related to morbidity (income lost from decreased productivity, restricted activity, and absenteeism) and mortality costs (the value of future income lost by premature death). There was a 197% increase in obesity-related hospitalizations among adolescents in the past 20 years, which has had a dire effect on the health care costs within this population (World Health Organization, 2003). The economic costs have also reached the school systems, where burdens related to students' absences cost districts between \$9 and \$20 per student (Action for Healthy Kids (AFHK), 2004). Since several states' funding was determined by attendance rates, the costs could be two-fold and should be considered a priority.

Table 1. Consequences of child and adolescent obesity

Types of consequences	
Physical	*Increased risk of developing:* Cardiovascular disease High blood pressure High cholesterol Type II diabetes Stroke Certain types of cancer Gallbladder disease Arthritis Sleep disturbances Asthma Maintain obesity into adulthood
Psychological	Depression Peer rejection Low self-esteem Feelings of shame and guilt Stigmatization Discrimination
Societal	Medical costs Morbidity costs Mortality costs School costs

Determinants of Overweight and Obesity

The factors which have contributed to overweight and obesity were considered numerous and complex. Body weight has been shaped by a combination of genetic, metabolic, behavioral, environmental, cultural, and socioeconomic influences. Some of the determinants are non-modifiable such as genetics, sex, age, and race. However, most of the population was more likely affected by the influences of surroundings, opportunities, or conditions predisposing individuals to obesity (Moreno et al., 2004).

The reason most often cited to cause obesity was related to an excess in energy consumption and/or inadequate physical activity (Office of the Surgeon General, 2001). Unhealthy eating and physical activity practices that contribute to childhood obesity tend to be established early in life; young persons having these unhealthy habits were likely to maintain them as they aged (CDC, 2005). Supported by the American Medical Association (Goutham, 2008), there were four well-recognized behaviors that have the capability of offsetting the development of childhood obesity (Table 2).

Therefore, when considering what will evoke change, the focus should be on those determinants which have been considered modifiable, prevalent, and relatively easy to target within children and adolescents. Again, during childhood and adolescence proved to be an important population, as behaviors which were related to obesity prevention declined during these years (Wilson, 2008).

Table 2. Modifiable behaviors related to childhood and adolescent obesity as recommended by the American Medical Association

Behaviors	
Physical Activity	Participation in at least 60 minutes of moderate to vigorous physical activity per day.
Sedentary Behaviors	Limiting screen time (television, video game, and computer use) to less than two hours per day.
Fruit and Vegetable Consumption	Eating five or more servings of fruit and vegetables daily.
Sweetened Beverage Consumption	Increasing water consumption in relation to the amount of sweetened beverages consumed.

Link between Nutrition and Health

The link between nutrition and health has been indicated time and time again. In order to achieve good health, an individual's nutritional choices become essential. Major causes of morbidity and mortality in the United States have been related to poor diet. Following a diet that complies with the Dietary Guidelines may reduce the risk of many of the chronic diseases associated with increased risk of morbidity and mortality (cardiovascular disease, hypertension, type 2 diabetes, osteoporosis, and some cancers) (USDHHS, 2005). It was estimated that about 16 % of mortality from any cause in men, and 9 % from any cause of mortality in women could be eliminated by the inclusion of recommended dietary behaviors (National Center for Education Statistics, 1996).

The link between nutrition and health for children and adolescents is of particular concern, as the relationship between their healthy growth and development has been indicated. The health of children and adolescents is dependent on obtaining food adequate in energy and nutrients to promote optimal physical, social, and cognitive growth and development (American Dietetic Association, 2006). Children and adolescents who do not meet these standards are at risk for a variety of poor outcomes, including growth retardation, iron deficiency anemia, poor academic performance, development of psychosocial difficulties, and an increased likelihood of developing the aforementioned chronic diseases. Not only has a link between delayed physical, psychosocial, and cognitive development been established, but the relationship between the growing problem of child and adolescent obesity cannot be ignored.

Benefits of a Health and Nutrition Education Curriculum

The benefits of a health and nutrition education curriculum were far reaching. Health and nutrition education have been known to help students with positive strides in their overall lifestyles, development of good personal habits, avoidance of high-risk behaviors, and with control over their own future (Merritt, 2008).

In fact, the American Dietetic Association (2005) has acknowledged the importance of nutrition education in their position statement:

> It is the position of the American Dietetic Association that all children and adolescents, regardless of age, sex, socioeconomic status, racial diversity, ethnic diversity, linguistic diversity, or health status, should have access to food and nutrition programs that ensure the availability of a safe and adequate food supply that promotes optimal physical, cognitive, social, and emotional growth and development. Appropriate food and nutrition programs include food assistance and meal programs, nutrition education initiatives, and nutrition screening and assessment followed by appropriate nutrition intervention and anticipatory guidance to promote optimal nutrition status.

With the mention of both "nutrition education initiatives" and "appropriate nutrition intervention" the American Dietetic Association (2006) has recognized that all children should be provided with the knowledge and skills necessary to make healthy nutrition choices. The importance of these strategies in reducing the prevalence of obesity among children and adolescents should be a main focus now and into the future.

Importance of Schools

Traditionally, one of the primary missions of schools has been to help children grow into healthy and productive adults (Merritt, 2008). Schools were considered an important venue for delivery of health education programs since a majority of the nation's youth can be reached (Goutham, 2008). In 2000, 53.2 million students were enrolled in public and private elementary and secondary schools in the United States (IOM, 2005). Children spent a majority of their hours in school, and all children regardless of demographics had the capability of being reached during school time. In addition, nutrition and physical activity behaviors were addressed in some capacity everyday through the choice of school meals, health and/or physical education curriculum (Procter et al., 2008). Schools also had other resources which increased the viability of school-based programming such as: classrooms, educational resources, educated individuals to supervise activities/programs, and access to additional health services including school nurses (Story, 1999). Furthermore, the school is an ideal environment when dealing with peer influence and social norm expectations in relation to eating behaviors related to obesity (Procter et al., 2008).

The existing educational mission of schools was suggested to be in line with the dissemination of health information (Pyle et al., 2006). However, today's schools have faced intense pressure to focus on standardized tests, and therefore have shifted away from an emphasis on a healthy mind and a healthy body (Wechsler, McKenna, Lee, & Dietz, 2004). An increasing number of educators have realized, as the National Association of State Boards of Education (NASBE) stated, "Health and success in school are interrelated. Schools cannot achieve their primary mission of educating if students and staff are not healthy and fit physically, mentally, and socially" (NASBE, 2000, p. 2). Schools can help to meet the goal of obesity reduction, i.e. healthier students, while boosting academic achievement and maintaining or improving their own financial situation (AFHK, 2004).

Both inside and outside of the classroom, schools present opportunities for students to learn about healthful eating habits and to make food choices during school meal times and through school-related activities (AFHK, 2004; IOM, 2005). Schools have been identified as important channels through which important behavior changes related to the reduction of childhood obesity could be addressed (Carter, Wiecha, Peterson, & Gortmaker, 2002; CDC, 1997; Wilson, 2008). School-based programs have also been found to be cost-effective (Wang, Yang, Lowry, & Wechsler, 2003). Hence, the Institute of Medicine (2005) in its *Preventing Childhood Obesity: Health in the Balance* report recommended that schools should provide a consistent environment that was conducive to healthful eating behaviors. School efforts to make policy and environmental changes have not gone unnoticed, however "It is not enough to change the food on the plate. We must also provide the knowledge and the skills that enable children to make choices that lead to a nutritious diet and improved health" (National Center for Education Statistics, 1996, p.2).

Students have also been receptive to the idea of school-based initiatives. When interviews were conducted with overweight students, they responded positively, given that the program would be presented in a supportive environment, was informative, and was tailored to their needs and concerns (Neumark-Sztainer, Martin & Story, 2000). A later study revealed similar findings, with additional suggestions for the program such as low cost, convenient, entertaining, inclusion of a variety of activities, and offered to all students regardless of their weight (Neumark-Sztainer, Story, & Martin, 2003). Wilson (2008) recommended the importance of incorporating what children and adolescents viewed as important into school-based nutrition education programs.

School Curriculum

Health and nutrition curriculum are incorporated in both the National Health Education Standards and the National Science Education Standards. In addition, there are also state health standards embedded in the curriculum, with most states having their own guidelines for curriculum and instruction (Merritt, 2008). It has been approximated that more than 80 percent of school districts in the U.S. are required to teach health education. However, the effectiveness of health education curricula has been faulted, as standards are not consistent across the board.

The general priorities in health instruction have included information on diet, eating disorders, and obesity prevention. More specifically, the following topics were constituted as "priorities" in nutrition education: children's food-related habits and eating behaviors; the relationship of food, diet and nutrients to health; the links between nutrition and cardiovascular health; the food-guide pyramid; finding and choosing healthy foods and increasing positive eating patterns; nutrients and their food sources; dietary guidelines and goals that emphasize low-fat, low-salt and increased complex-carbohydrate foods. Within these topics, curriculum must be developmentally appropriate. Table 3 summarizes the main nutrition curricular concepts underlying grade-specific National Science Education Standards.

Table 3. National Science-Education Standards – Nutrition

Curricular Area: Nutrition	Statement of Curricular Concept/Principle
Grades K-4	Nutrition is essential to health. Students should understand how the body uses food and how various foods contribute to health. Recommendations for good nutrition include eating a variety of foods, eating less sugar and eating less fat.
Grades 5-8	Food provides energy and nutrients for growth and development. Nutrition requirements vary with body weight, age, sex, activity and body functioning.
Grades 9-12	Selection of foods and eating patterns determine nutritional balance. Nutritional balance has a direct effect on growth, development and personal well-being. Personal and social factors – such as habits, family income, ethnic heritage, body size, advertising and peer pressure – influence nutritional choices.

Review of Nutrition Education School-Based Obesity Prevention Programs

Lessons need to be learned from past, present and future programs which include nutrition education as a means to prevent obesity in children and adolescents. In settings where time, teacher preparation, cost, student attention span, and limited resources are constraints, measuring the effectiveness of such programs becomes imperative (Abood, Black & Coster, 2008). Several reviews have been conducted which highlight the vast array of nutrition education programming being included in school-based obesity prevention programs. See Table 4 for a summary of these interventions.

Table 4. Summary of nutrition education programs

Program/ Author	Purpose	Theory	Sample	Description of Program/ Nutrition Component	Major Findings	Author Suggestions
Choice, Control & Change Contento et al., 2007	To encourage personal agency and competence in both nutrition and physical activity behaviors.	TPB	Middle school students in 19 science classes within 5 schools (n=278)	24-sessions The curriculum used a unique inquiry-based scientific approach.	Students increased consumption of fruits and vegetables, decreased the frequency of sweetened beverages, packaged snacks, and eating at fast food restaurants.	Through this approach, students developed an in-depth understanding of the rationale for taking action, and the expected barriers, an increase in self-efficacy, and a sense of empowerment.

Table 4. (Continued)

Program/ Author	Purpose	Theory	Sample	Description of Program/ Nutrition Component	Major Findings	Author Suggestions
Fit For Life Gombosi et al., 2007	To investigate a primary obesity prevention program focusing on both nutrition and physical activity as a way to a healthier lifestyle, also recognizing the importance of family and community.		Students in grades K-8 and their families. (n = 4241 ± 200/year)	American Heart Association kits provided to nearly all classrooms. The Virtual Reality Wellness Club, a series of work booklets that progressively challenge participants to track their physical activity and nutrition choices.	Outcome data did not show significant improvement in knowledge or BMI outcomes.	Helped enhance the use of a standard health curriculum.
Frenn's Study Frenn et al., 2003	To reduce fat intake in diet and increase physical activity in middle school students.	Health Promot-ion Model, TM	6th – 8th grade, experimental group (n = 60) and control (n = 57)	4 classroom 45-min. sessions based on stage of change Focus on consciousness raising and self-reevaluation. Use of age-specific examples, games, preparation and sampling of snacks.	Percentage fat in food was sig. less and duration of exercise for intervention group was sig. higher.	Short interventions might be viable options in the right setting.
Louisiana Health Williamson et al., 2008	To modify environment al cues, enhance social support, and promote self-efficacy for health behavior change.	SCT	17 school clusters assigned to one of three intervention arms (n = 775, 727, 600)	Program delivered as part of regular classroom instruction, combined with internet counseling and email communications for children and their parents. Children will receive weekly lessons on healthy eating and exercise that include a 20–25 min interactive didactic segment followed by hands-on activities.	Results to come.	The target population represent poor families who could not readily access appropriate health care or preventive services.

Table 4. (Continued)

Program/ Author	Purpose	Theory	Sample	Description of Program/ Nutrition Component	Major Findings	Author Suggestions
Michigan Model Nutrition Curriculum Fahlman et al., 2008	To determine the impact of the curriculum on nutrition knowledge, efficacy expectations, and eating behaviors.		Middle school students divided into an intervention group (n = 407) and a control group (n = 169).	Teachers were trained to incorporate the 8 lessons into their curriculum. Topics related to nutrition knowledge such as the food groups, food pyramid, food labels, advertising, and body image. They also contained components specifically designed to target nutritional risk behaviors.	In the intervention group: increased nutrition knowledge, significantly more likely to eat FV and less likely to eat junk food, and felt more confident that they could eat healthy.	Well-designed and -executed school-based nutrition programs can result in positive changes in dietary eating behaviors, as well as increased self-efficacy expectancy regarding nutritional choices in middle school children. Further research needed to determine the long-term impact.
New Moves Neumark-Stainer et al., 2003 Flattum et al., 2009	To increase physical activity, healthful eating, and social support when implemented as a multi-component, girls-only PE class.	SCT	14-17 yr. old inactive adolescent high school girls (n = 41)	16-week program (once every other week) Focused on skill building and self-efficacy through use of small groups, class discussions, role play, preparing and eating healthy snacks. Follow-up sessions included individual sessions, using motivational interviewing to develop goals and actions related to eating and physical activity.	Majority of initial outcomes were not significant. Among the 20 girls who were a part of the motivational interviewing, 81% completed all of the individual sessions, and girls set a goal 100% of the time.	Gender specific education may help those who face barriers in traditional co-ed classes. Motivational interviewing offers a promising component of school-based obesity-prevention programs and was found to be feasible to implement in school settings and acceptable to the adolescents.

Table 4. (Continued)

Program/ Author	Purpose	Theory	Sample	Description of Program/ Nutrition Component	Major Findings	Author Suggestions
Nutrition in the Garden McAleese & Rankin, 2007	To investigate the effects of garden-based nutrition education on adolescents' fruit and vegetable consumption.		Sixth grade students (n=99) at three different elementary schools made up a control and two treatment groups.	The 12-week curriculum provided lessons and activities that combined nutrition and hands-on, garden-based activities. Students were also involved in food experiences with FV harvested from the garden.	Adolescents who participated in the garden-based nutrition intervention increased their servings of FV more than students in the two other groups.	These results help to show the importance of hands-on activities when attempting to change nutrition-related behavior such as fruit and vegetable consumption.
Pathways Caballero et al., 2003	To evaluate the effectiveness of a school-based multi-component intervention for reducing body fat in American Indian children including classroom curriculum, food service modifications, physical activity and family involvement.	SCT	3rd – 5th grade (n = 1,704)	12-weeks (2 x 45-min. lessons) Classroom curriculum was based on relevant culture and practices.	Knowledge, attitudes and behaviors were positively and sig. changed.	Curricular changes can improve knowledge and behaviors. Longer interventions may be needed to see sig. changes in percent body fat.
Pilot Community Prevention Program Hawley et al., 2008	To educate students and families about the importance of good nutrition and exercise and to motivate them to reach these goals by using principles of behavior change.	TM	Sixth graders (n = 65) and their families	The program consisted of five 40-min sessions during physical education classes, over the course of 6 weeks. Instruction was in nutrition, fitness, goal setting, and self-efficacy. Sessions consisted of adventure-based games and tasks. A family component helped get students started and focused on setting and working towards goals.	There were no sig changes in students' individual health attitudes and behaviors. However, sig changes did occur among families -the goal of eating healthfully was sig more important.	The preliminary study provided a strong foundation on which to build an intervention that addressed the community's particular nutrition and activity challenges.

Table 4. (Continued)

Program/ Author	Purpose	Theory	Sample	Description of Program/ Nutrition Component	Major Findings	Author Suggestions
Planet Health Gortmaker et al., 1999	To integrate the health goals of increasing physical activity, decreasing TV viewing, improving FV intake, and moderating fat intake into the middle school curriculum.	SCT	6th – 8th grade, implemented with 129 teachers in 6 schools	32 classroom lessons integrated into other disciplines	Reduced obesity in girls, increased FV consumption, reduced TV watching.	Found to be feasible and acceptable when implemented in the school setting.
Policy-based school intervention Foster et al., 2008	To examine the effects of a multi-component, school nutrition policy initiative; and show how food choices and physical activity are tied to personal behavior, individual health, and the environment.		Participants were 1349 students in 4th – 6th grade from 10 schools with 50% of students eligible for free or reduced-price meals.	The goal was to integrate nutrition (50 hours/year) into various disciplines. The educational component was designed to be integrative and interdisciplinary.	There was a 50% reduction in the incidence of overweight. Significantly fewer children in the intervention schools (7.5%) than in the control schools (14.9%) became overweight after 2 years.	A multicomponent school-based intervention can be effective in preventing the development of overweight.
Present and Prevent Abood et al., 2008	To assess a school-based nutrition minimal intervention which used a commercially available power-point program.		Middle school students (mean age = 14.5), experimental group (n = 551), delayed treatment group (n = 329)	Program presented in two 30-minute time slots over 1 week. Included information on : health problems associated with and causes of obesity, importance of preventing obesity, body image, benefits of and achieving healthy body weight, healthful food choices, reading food labels, portion control, how to	Significant experimental improvement occurred in: knowledge, intention to maintain a healthy body weight because of importance to friends, intention to eat fewer fried foods, eat fewer sweets, look more at food labels, and limit TV watching.	The impact of the minimal program should be considered with decreased school resources, as well as the attention span and interest level of teens. Nutrition education MIs may serve as an adjunct to existing approaches to obesity

Table 4. (Continued)

Program/ Author	Purpose	Theory	Sample	Description of Program/ Nutrition Component	Major Findings	Author Suggestions
				change unhealthful habits, how to start being more active and overcoming barriers.		prevention
USDA fresh fruit and vegetable program Jamelske et al., 2008	Whether an impact was made by the FFVP, which provided funding for students to receive a free fresh fruit or vegetable snack daily for an academic year.		4th, 7th, and 9th graders (n = 1127) 784 students in 10 intervention schools and 343 students in 10 control schools	Students were provided with fruit and vegetable snacks daily for a year to see if exposure to different fruits and vegetables would alter attitudes, behaviors.	Intervention students reported an increased willingness to try new fruits (24.8% versus 12.8%) and vegetables (25.1% versus 18.4%) at school.	Consumption of FV as a habit in childhood is an important predictor of higher consumption as adults. It is essential that the effects of school, district, or state policy changes regarding the school food environment are evaluated.
Ward-Begnoche et al., 2008	To incorporate nutritional, physical activity, and coping skills curriculum that emphasized education and behavioral change into the PE curriculum.		Middle school students (6th – 8th grade) taking physical education (n = 78)	16-sessions including worksheets, handouts, and structured activities. Small group format was used to aid in rapport building with instructors. Information included food labels, review of popular fast food restaurants' nutritional information, and portion size.	Results to come.	Benefits identified included helping the school to establish a nutrition and physical activity goal for their school, provide teachers and personnel an opportunity to facilitate goal-setting and behavior-change curriculum.

Components of Successful Programs

As several reviews have indicated, implementing nutrition education programs in the school does not necessarily ensure success. However, these reviews have also shown common components amongst successful programs (Table 5). The inclusion of all three components: the cognitive, the affective (conative) and the behavioral (volitional) has led to numerous successful nutrition education programs (Contento, Balch, & Bronner, 1995). The cognitive component focuses on providing factual nutrition information. The affective component includes beliefs, attitudes, and perceptions associated with healthy nutrition behaviors. The behavioral component supports the change process, goal-setting, skill building and readiness. Lessons have been learned within each of these components and should be considered when designing successful nutrition education obesity prevention programs in the school setting. In addition, programs complemented with physical activity were more successful in altering BMI outcomes.

Nutrition education programs which promoted healthy weight rather than focusing on weight loss or attaining a specific weight were less likely to intensify diet and self-reported insecurities (Pyle et al., 2006). It was recommended for programs to focus on improving nutrition habits in combination with physical activity, and other healthy lifestyle choices.

Table 5. Components of successful nutrition education programs

Behavioral focus
Theoretical framework
Adequate time and intensity
Family involvement
Multicomponent strategies
Developmentally appropriate
Considers needs of students, teachers and school
Strengthen self-efficacy, skills
Culturally relevant
Evaluation

An essential component of these nutrition education programs, either primary or secondary, was a focus on behavior change (Caballero, 2004). Most successful programs combined several different techniques including: behavior management counseling, teaching strategies to identify healthy foods and avoid unhealthy foods, implementing healthy nutritional choices into the daily menu, and involving parents and other family members throughout the program (Pyle et al., 2006). To be effective, programs should focus on promoting healthy behaviors in a way to impact consequent behavior into and throughout adulthood.

Nutrition education was an integral element within successful child and adolescent school-based obesity prevention programs. Providing age-appropriate, culturally sensitive instruction and materials was connected to the positive behavioral outcomes of the programs (AFHK, 2004). Effective programs in diverse communities must be especially cognicent of individuals and their backgrounds, and tailor the programs as such (Perez-Rodrigo & Aranceta, 2003). Casazza and Ciccazzo (2006) indicated the effectiveness of a nutrition-education program when relevant to the student, as well as the applicability of the information to the student's everyday life. Focusing on learning styles of "today's" children and adolescents becomes vital. Computer-based, interactive, animated education programs were effective in eliciting nutrition behavior changes.

To adopt, maintain, and enjoy healthy nutrition habits it is critical to go beyond dissemination of knowledge and to promote the development of attitudes, skills, and behaviors. Use of behavioral theories often help in going beyond simple dissemination of knowledge. Examples of behavioral theories are: health belief model, social cognitive theory, transtheoretical model, theory of reasoned action, and theory of planned behavior. McAleese, Rankin and Fada (2007) established the importance of hands-on activities, such as schoolyard gardens, when attempting to change nutrition-related behaviors. McAleese et al. (2007) found children and adolescent to be more receptive when they were involved with a project related to their desired nutrition goals.

However, in such programs nutrition education also went further than the expected classroom education. Schools have been described as having the opportunity to influence the nutrition children receive, as well as helping to establish healthy lifelong habits by including school personnel in modeling healthy choices; advocating for healthy eating by providing healthy school lunches and snacks; exposing students to the selection, preparation, and taste of healthful foods (Pyle et al., 2006). Since nearly every school in the nation served at least one meal a day, five days a week, the impact of these changes, coupled with effective nutrition education could be immense (Haskins, Paxson, & Donahue, 2006).

Challenges of Nutrition Education in School-based Programs

Although schools seem to be an ideal setting to implement nutrition education programs which could contribute to obesity prevention, there are challenges which present roadblocks to implementation. Increasing curricular mandates, time demands on teachers, and financial strain on the school systems have all contributed to the decreased importance placed on health education, including nutrition education, within the school curriculum (Merritt, 2008). Many times these subjects are overlooked or taught briefly within other subjects, thereby decreasing the effectiveness of learning.

The ever-changing diverse student body also presents a challenge to the implementation of nutrition education programs (Merritt, 2008). Many students come from very different backgrounds, including differences in race/ethnicity, cultural beliefs, socioeconomic status, and parental involvement just to name a few. With recommendations hinging on the information presented being relevant to the student, this creates some challenges.

Parental buy-in plays a role in the efficacy of nutrition education programs. Unfortunately most parents do not set good examples for their children. Without the inclusion and responsiveness of parents, the educational messages taught throughout the nutrition program may be lost (Merritt, 2008).

Adequate training to teach the nutrition education programs has often been overlooked. In order for teachers to teach the curricula effectively, they must be properly trained (Merritt, 2008). This typically involves time and money which the school systems do not have. Having a support person for such a program also tends to help the implementation, as well as the sustainability of the program. Most schools do not have funds allocated for such a position, leaving the coordination of said program up in the air.

Recommendations for School-based Nutrition Education Interventions

With such a huge focus on childhood obesity, numerous leaders in health education have proposed recommendations to improve the success of school-based programs. The Institute of Medicine (2005) realized that teaching children the importance of health promotion practices was a priority and school was considered an ideal place for promoting habits that would support a healthy future. The IOM suggested schools must take the opportunity to provide lessons in healthy behaviors that will allow children to be more effective learners, as well as provide a consistent environment conducive to healthful eating behaviors. In order for this to happen, schools should be provided with adequate and sustained federal and state government funding to implement changes in the school environment and provide appropriate nutrition education (IOM, 2006).

School environmental factors included improved school health curricula (with innovative approaches to teaching and staffing); school health services for obesity prevention efforts; school meals that met the Dietary Guidelines for Americans; nutritional standards for all competitive foods and beverages sold or served in schools (IOM, 2006). In addition, it was recommended that schools conduct an annual assessment of students' weight, height, and body mass index and make the information available to parents in an effort to identify at-risk children.

In addition to the school environment, personal, behavioral, social and community environmental factors must be considered. School-based nutrition education programs should consider the needs and interests of students, teachers, and the school (Perez-Rodrigo & Aranceta, 2003). As reported in a review by Doak et al. (2006), effective programs need to be tailored to the individual needs of the children, according to gender and ethnicity. Future interventions should also address the psychological and environmental influences of the home environment through education and active involvement of parents. Developing partnerships with parents and communities would allow schools to fight childhood obesity more effectively and ensure a healthy future for the children (IOM, 2005; Rosenthal & Chang, 2004).

Beyond the content of the nutrition education programs, it was noted that obesity prevention messages should be framed positively. Focusing on potential solutions rather than on problems was more likely to cause people to take action. The relationship between children's emotional well-being in relation to overweight and obesity was not assessed in most programs. Doak et al. (2006) warned that singling out children at risk may contribute to their emotional and mental distress. The impact of the children's emotional well-being indicated the need to further explore not only the specific messages being targeted, but also the delivery and implementation of the program.

CDC Recommendations. The Centers for Disease Control and Prevention (CDC, 1997) published guidelines that identified school policies and practices most likely to be effective in promoting lifelong physical activity and healthy eating. The guidelines were directly related to many of the recommendations for school-based interventions. As such, the CDC recommendations should be considered important when initiating nutrition-related changes in school environments and programming. The guidelines applicable to school-based nutrition education programs are as follows: 1) address nutrition through a Coordinated School Health Program (CSHP) approach; 2) designate a school health coordinator and maintain an active school health council; 3) assess the school's health policies and programs and develop a plan for improvement; 4) strengthen the school's nutrition policies; 5) implement a high-quality health promotion program for school staff; 6) implement a high-quality course of study in health education; 7) implement a quality school meals program; and 8) ensure that students have appealing, healthy choices in foods and beverages offered outside of the school meals program.

Research has shown that in schools where nutrition education efforts are coordinated, a more focused message about the importance of healthy eating is presented. Integration across the curriculum and building on lessons from year to year can only enhance the success of nutrition education programs in the school setting (National Center for Education Statistics, 1996).

CONCLUSION

The need for improved nutrition among America's youth is evident, as the rates of child and adolescent overweight and obesity continue to increase. The complexity of the issue has made a solution difficult. It is understood that schools cannot solve the obesity epidemic on their own (Wechsler et al., 2000), but school-based nutrition education programs have the potential for reaching numerous children in a cost-effective manner (Plye et al., 2006). The former U.S. Surgeon General has been quoted as saying, "I do not blame schools for our obesity epidemic. Instead I look to schools – and everyone who has an influential hand in education – as a powerful force for change" (Office of the Surgeon General, 2001). Skills taught in school-based programs are accepted as the foundations for healthy lifestyles, regardless of children's weight status. As expressed by those involved with Action for Healthy Kids, providing the resources and tools which evoke change was a necessity. Just as the problems which have led to obesity were multifaceted, the solutions need to be as well (AFHK, 2004).

Development of healthy lifestyle habits that persist into adulthood, and thus, have a long-term impact on the health and well-being of future generations is critical (USDHHS, 2007). The diversity of nutrition education programs which have been effective has been promising: the likelihood of finding a suitable program, adaptable to specific community needs is upon us (Doak et al., 2006). Nevertheless, nutrition education programs must be developed around community needs, and guided by those which have already been successful. As Doak et al. stated, "There is no need to reinvent the wheel" (p.129). Building on successful programs and relating them to the child, adolescent, and specific community needs will increase the likelihood of success. These significant lessons must be used to make an impact on the childhood obesity epidemic which continues to plague our nation.

REFERENCES

Abood, D., Black, D. & Coster, D. (2008). Evaluation of a school-based teen obesity prevention minimal intervention. *Journal of Nutrition Education and Behavior, 40,* 168-174.

Action for Healthy Kids. (2004). *The value of improving nutrition and physical activity in our schools.* Retrieved July 9, 2008 from www.actionforhealthykids.org

American Dietetic Association. (2006). Position of the American Dietetic Association: Child and adolescent food and nutrition programs. *Journal of the American Dietetic Association, 106,* 1467-1475.

Caballero, B., Clay, T., Davis, S., Ethelbath, B., Rock, B., Lohman, T., et al. (2003). Pathways: A school-based randomized controlled trial for the prevention of obesity in American Indian school children. *American Journal of Clinical Nutrition, 78,* 1030-1038.

Caballero, B. (2004). Obesity prevention in children: Opportunities and challenges. *Journal of Obesity, 28,* S90-S95.

Carter, J., Wiecha, J., Peterson, K. & Gormaker, S. (2001). *An interdisciplinary curriculum for teaching middle school nutrition and physical activity.* Champaign, IL: Human Kinetics.

Casazza, K., & Ciccazzo, M. (2006). Improving the dietary patterns of adolescents using a computer-based approach. *Journal of School Health, 76,* 43-46.

Centers for Disease Control and Prevention. (1997). Guidelines for school and community programs to promote lifelong physical activity among young people. *MMWR, 46,* 1-36.

Centers for Disease Control and Prevention, National Center for Health Statistics. (2005). *National health and nutrition examination survey (NHANES).* Retrieved October 10,2007 from http: www.cdc.gov/nchs/about/major/nhanes/nhanes2005-2006/nhanes05_06.html

Contento, I., Balch, G., & Bronner, Y. (1995). Theoretical frameworks of models for nutrition education. *Journal of Nutrition Education, 27,* 287-290.

Contento, I., Koch, P., Lee, H., Sauberli, W. & Calabrese-Barton, A. (2007). Enhancing personal agency and competence in eating and moving: Formative evaluations of a middle school curriculum – Choice, control, and change. *Journal of Nutrition Education Behavior, 39,* 179-186.

Cooley, C. (1964). *Human nature and the social order.* New York: Schocken.

Cosrow, N., Jeffrey, R., & McGuire, M. (2001). Understanding weight stigmatization: A focus group study. *Journal of Nutrition Education, 33,* 208-214.

Doak, C. M., Visscher, T., Renders, M. & Seidell, J. C. (2006). The prevention of overweight and obesity in children and adolescents: A review of interventions and programmes. *Obesity Reviews, 7,* 111-136.

Erickson, S., Robinson, T., Haydel, K. & Killen, J. (2000). Are overweight children unhappy. *Archives of Pediatrics and Adolescent Medicine, 154,* 931-934.

Evans, W., Finkelstein, E., Kamerow, D., & Renaud, J. (2005). Public perceptions of childhood obesity. *American Journal of Preventive Medicine, 28,* 26-32.

Fahlman, M., Dake, J., McCaughtry, N., & Martin, J. (2008). A pilot study to examine the effects of a nutrition intervention on nutrition knowledge, behaviors, and efficacy expectations in middle school children. *Journal of School Health, 78,* 216-222.

Finkelstein, E., Fiebelkorn, I., Wang, G. (2003). National medical spending attributable to overweight and obesity: How much, and who's paying? *Health Affairs, 3,* 219–226.

Flattum, C., Friend, S., Neumark-Sztainer, D., & Story, M. (2009). Motivational interviewing as a component of a school-based obesity prevention program for adolescent girls. *Journal of American Dietetic Association, 109,* 91-94.

Foster, G., Sherman, S., Borradalie, K., Grudny, K., Vander Veur, S., Nahcmani, J., et al. (2008). A policy-based school intervention to prevent overweight and obesity. *Pediatrics, 121,* 794-802.

Freedman, D. S., Dietz, W. H., Srinivasan, S. R. & Berenson, G. S. (1999). The relation of overweight to cardiovascular risk factors among children and adolescents: The Bogalusa

Frenn, M., Malin, S. & Bansal, N. (2003). Stage-based intervention for low-fat diet with middle school students. *Journal of Pediatric Nursing, 18,* 36-45.

Gombosi, R., Olasin, R. & Bittle, J. (2007). Tioga county fit for life: A primary obesity prevention project. *Clinical Pediatrics, 46,* 592-600.

Gortmaker, S., Peterson, Wiecha, J., Sobaol, A., Dixit, S., Fox, M. & Laird, N. (1999). Reducing obesity via school-based interdisciplinary intervention among youth: Planet Health. *Archives of Pediatric Adolescent Medicine, 153,* 409-418.

Goutham, R. (2008). Childhood obesity: Highlights of AMA expert committee recommendations. *American Family Physician, 78,* 56-64.

Haskins, R., Paxson, C., & Donahue, E. (2006). *Future of children: Fighting obesity in the public schools.* Princeton Brookings. Retrieved July 9, 2008 from www.futreofchildren.org

Hawley, S., Beckman, H. & Bishop, T. (2006). Development of an obesity prevention and management program for children and adolescents in a rural setting. *Journal of Community Health Nursing, 23,* 69-80.

Heart Study. *Pediatrics, 103,* 1175-1182.

Institute of Medicine. (2004). *Preventing childhood obesity: Health in the balance.* Washington, DC: National Academy Press.

Institute of Medicine. (2005). *Preventing Childhood Obesity: Health in the Balance.* Retrieved July 9, 2008 from www.iom.edu

Institute of Medicine (2006). *Progress in Preventing Childhood Obesity: How Do We Measure Up?* Washington, DC: National Academies Press, Retrieved July 9, 2008 from www.nap.edu

Jamelske, E., Bica, L., McCarty, D. & Meinen, A. (2008). Preliminary findings from an evaluation of the USDA fresh fruit and vegetable program in Wisconsin schools. *Wisconsin Medical Journal, 107,* 225-230.

Kaufman, F. R. (2003). Type 2 diabetes in children and youth. *Reviews in Endocrine & Metabolic Disorders, 4,* 33-42.

Lobstein, T., Baur, L., Uauy, R. & International Association for the Study of Obesity Task Force. (2004). Obesity in children and young people: A crisis in public health. *Obesity Reviews, 5*(Suppl. 1), 4-104.

McAleese, J. & Rankin, L. (2007). Garden-based nutrition education affects fruit and vegetable consumption in sixth-grade adolescents. *Journal of the American Dietetic Association, 107,* 662-665.

Merritt, R. D. (2008). Health and nutrition studies: Curriculum organization – Health and nutrition in the curriculum. Research Starters: EBSCO Publishing Inc.

Moreno, L. A., Tomas, C., Gonzalez-Gross, M., Bueno, G., Perez-Gonzalez, J. M. & Bueno, M. (2004). Micro-environmental and socio-demographic determinants of childhood obesity. *International Journal of Obesity and Related Metabolic Disorders, 28* (Suppl. 3), S16-S20.

National Association of State Boards of Education. (2000). *Fit, healthy, and ready to learn.* Alexandria, VA: Author.

National Center for Education Statistics. (1996). Nutrition education in public elementary and secondary schools.

Neumark-Sztainer, D., Martin, S.L. & Story, M. (2000). School-based programs for obesity prevention: What do adolescents recommend? *American Journal of Health Promotion, 14,* 232–235.

Neumark-Sztainer, D., Story, M. & Martin, S. (2003). New moves: A school-based obesity prevention program for adolescent girls. *Preventive Medicine, 37,* 41-51.

Office of the Surgeon General. (2001). *The Surgeon General's call to action to prevent and decrease overweight and obesity*. Rockville, MD: Author.

Ogden, C. L., Flegal, K. M., Carroll, M. D. & Johnson, C. L. (2002). Prevalence and trends in overweight among U.S. children and adolescents, 1999-2000. *Journal of the American Medical Association, 288,* 1728-1732.

Perez-Rodrigo, C. & Aranceta, J. (2003). Nutrition education in schools: Experiences and challenges. *European Journal of Clinical Nutrition, 57,* S82-S85.

Procter, K. L., Rudolf, M. C., Feltbower, R. G., Levine, R., Connor, A., Robinson, M. et al. (2008). Measuring the school impact on child obesity. *Social Science and Medicine, 67,* 341-349.

Pyle, S., Sharkey, J., Yetter, G., Felix, E. & Furlong, M. (2006). Fighting an epidemic: The role of schools in reducing childhood obesity. *Psychology in the School, 43,* 361-375.

Rosenthal, J. & Chang, D. (2004). *State approaches to childhood obesity: A snapshot of promising practices and lessons learned.* National Academy for State Health Policy: Portland, ME.

Schwartz, M. & Puhl, R. (2003). Childhood obesity: A societal problem to solve. *Obesity Reviews, 4,* 57-71.

Schwimmer, J., Burwinkle, T. & Varni, J. (2003). Health-related quality of life of severely obese children and adolescents. *The Journal of the American Medical Association, 289,* 1813-1819.

Shelton. (2008). Physicians increasingly seeing overweight children with "adult" diseases. *Chicago Tribune, 3/19/08.*

Smith, J. (2004). The current epidemic of childhood obesity and its implications for future coronary heart disease. *Pediatric Clinics of North America, 51,* 1679-1695.

Story, M. (1999). School-based approaches for preventing and treating obesity. *International Journal of Obesity, 23,* S43-S51.

Strauss, R. S. (2000). Childhood obesity and self esteem. *Pediatrics, 105*, E15.

U.S. Department of Health and Human Services. (2004). *Prevalence of overweight among children and adolescents: United States 2003-2004*. Atlanta, GA:

U.S. Department of Health and Human Services, Centers for Disease Control and Prevention. Retrieved March 1, 2009 from http://www.cdc.gov/nchs/products/pubs/pubd/ hestats/ overweight/overwght_child_03.htm

U.S. Department of Health and Human Services & U.S. Department of Agriculture. (2005). *Dietary Guidelines for Americans*, 2005 (6th Edition). Washington, DC: U.S. Government Printing Office.

U.S. Department of Health and Human Services. (2007). *Overweight and obesity*. U.S. Department of Health and Human Services, Centers for Disease Control and Prevention. Retrieved March 1, 2009 from http://www.cdc.gov/nccdphp/dnpa/obesity/childhood/index.htm

Wang, L., Yang, Q., Lowry, R. & Wechsler, H. (2003). Economic analysis of a school-based obesity prevention program. *Obesity Research, 11,* 1313-1324.

Ward-Begnoche, W., Gance-Cleveland, B., Harris, M. & Dean, J. (2008). Description of the design and implementation of a school-based obesity prevention program addressing needs of middle school students. *Journal of Applied Clinical Psychology, 24,* 247-263.

Wechsler, H., McKenna, M., Lee, S. & Dietz, W. (2004). The role of schools in preventing childhood obesity. *The State Education Standard, December, 4-12.*

Whitaker, R., Wright, J., Pepe, M., Seidel, K. & Dietz, W. (1997). Predicting obesity in young adulthood from childhood and parental obesity. *New England Journal of Medicine, 337,* 467-474.

Williamson, D., Champagne, C., Harsha, D., Han, H., Martin, C., Newton, R., et al. (2008). Louisiana (LA) health: Design and methods for a childhood obesity prevention program in rural schools. *Contemporary Clinical Trials, 29,* 783-795.

Wilson, L. (2008). Adolescents' attitudes about obesity and what they want in obesity prevention programs. *The Journal of School Nursing, 23,* 229-238.

World Health Organization (2003). Obesity and overweight, 2003. Retrieved March 1, 2009 from http://www.who.int/dietphysicalactivity/publications/facts/obesity/en/print.html

In: Nutritional Education
Editor: Ida R. Laidyth

ISBN: 978-1-60876-078-7

Chapter 4

Human Sexual Dimorphism Underlying Gene-by- Nutrient Interaction

M. J. Mosher and M. H. Crawford*
Lab of Biological Anthropology, University of Kansas, KS, USA

Abstract

Nutrition plays both an ongoing and fluctuating environmental role influencing gene expression and observed phenotypic variation of complex traits, such as the serum lipid transport system. Individual nutritional status is influenced by a mélange of multiple cultural, biological, generational, epigenetic and genetic factors, all of which can ultimately affect the genetic profiles of a population. Despite increasing awareness of sex-specific effects, few research studies address the mechanisms by which factors of sexual dimorphism may influence the relationship between nutrients and genes in trait expression. Not all differences can be solely attributed to the direct effect of sex hormones. The effects of body composition, metabolically active adipose tissue and its active adipokines, macronutrient energy preference and metabolism are among the potential underlying factors affecting normal sex-specific expression of nutrient-by-gene interaction on complex traits. This chapter explores the mechanisms through which both direct and indirect effects of steroid hormones may influence biomarkers of lipid metabolism. Given the emphasis on dietary manipulation of serum lipids as a primary strategy in prevention of cardiovascular disease (CVD), further research addressing aspects of sexual dimorphism underlying variation of the lipid profile is imperative.

We examine current literature addressing the effects of nutrition and sexual dimorphism in body composition, fat patterning and hormones, energy homeostasis and metabolism and their association with serum lipids. Studies of dietary strategies as the first line of defense against susceptibility to disease have often concentrated on male subjects, with little understanding of female variation, and therefore having inconsistent results when applied to females.

* Corresponding author: mjmosher@aol.com

INTRODUCTION

The relationship between human energy homeostasis, lipid metabolism, and cholesterol is complex. Nutritional effects begin *in utero*, are ongoing, and context specific, while responsive to diet, sex, age, exercise status, female menstrual phase, body composition, and metabolically active adipose tissue. [Rees et al, 2008]. The steroid sex hormones of estrogen, progesterone and testosterone are present in both sexes, with their levels of concentration decidedly sex-specific. These hormones are synthesized from cholesterol, the lipid acquired through lipoprotein transport to the gonads and adrenals or synthesized directly in these glands from acetate [Braunstein, 1994; Goldfien and Monroe, 1994]. All hormones have widespread direct and indirect effects on many traits underlying sexual dimorphism in energy homeostasis and metabolism [Tarnopolsky, 1999]. Despite the surfeit of animal research showing significant evidence of dimorphism in metabolically active adipose tissue, substrate preference and metabolism, there is a paucity of substantial human studies which simultaneously examine both male and female samples. Unfortunately, many papers relating new findings in human biology and physiology make no reference to sex-differences, giving an impression that 'one explanation fits all'. This is simply not the case [Wizemann and Pardue, 2001]. In this chapter, we review current literature regarding normal human sexual dimorphism in the interrelated components of body composition, energy homeostasis and nutrition, with an emphasis on their effects on the lipid transport system. We select papers which consider both sexes together and sexual dimorphism specifically. Studies dealing with normal variation in physiology are stressed, while not emphasizing pathologies such as metabolic syndrome, diabetes or obesity

Lipid transport and metabolism are accomplished through series of interconnected bioactive pathways, whose components include fats and cholesterol (lipids), lipoproteins, apoproteins, enzymes, binding proteins and cell-surface receptors [Weiss 1993; Corella and Ordovas, 2005]. Beyond functioning as an energy source, lipids are vital to the human body through: 1) hedgehog protein activation and fetal programming [Woollett, 2008; Rees et al, 2008]; 2) cell membrane construction and modulation of dynamics; 3) structural precursors to steroid hormones and 4) energy and calcium homeostasis and inflammatory process mediation [Wenk, 2005]. Elements of the transport system components are often used as biomarkers to assess an individual's regulation of lipid metabolism and disease risk profiles. Unraveling the architecture underlying these lipid biomarkers is highly complex, given that similar phenotypes may actually arise from different genotypes, environments and the interaction of these factors [Weiss, 1993].

Once widely accepted as prevention and early intervention strategy against dyslipidemias and their sequelae of cardiovascular disease, dietary manipulation of serum lipid biomarkers is now under scrutiny [Werkö, 2008: Weinberg, 2004]. The absence of consistent response to conventional dietary adjustments suggests that underlying genetic variation may impact dietary affects. Studies comparing genotypes of selected candidate genes and their variation in dietary response produce few consistent results [Weggemans et al, 2001] and may be due to small effects, small sample sizes, retrospective study design [Masson et al, 2003], differences in environmental context-- such as age, and ethnicity [Ye and Kwiterovich, 2000; Corella and Ordovas, 2005], or by pooling males and females together --producing results that simply do not reflect either sex accurately [Stengard et al, 2002]. Early studies reported dietary effects on dyslipidemia were not as effective in females as in males [Ernst, 1980], and complicated by variation in female response associated to specific hormonal status [Legato, 1997]. Genes selected for maximum survival during times of starvation coupled with the reproductive responsibilities of the female to maintain a uterine environment conducive to fetal growth and development [Adair and Prentice, 2004], may, in fact, provide clues for explaining some inconsistencies currently described in gene by diet interaction underlying metabolism and lipid profiles.

Over sixty known genes are implicated in lipid metabolism, with others showing significant associations not yet replicated in subsequent studies [Corella and Ordovas, 2005]. Sex-specific quantitative trait loci (QTL) underlying lipoprotein variation have been suggested by several genome-wide linkage studies [Mosher et al, 2005; Weiss, et al, 2006]. Sex-by-gene variation in lipid concentrations have been recently reported [Senti,et al, 2002; Qi et al, 2004; Frikke-Schmidt et al, 2004; Hubacek et al, 2008; Talmud et al, 2001], including a sex-by-gene-by nutrient interaction [Mothered al., 2008]. A recent publication by Patsopoulos, et al. challenged gene by sex differences in 77 articles, claiming that many of these reports were spurious or poorly documented. These authors recommended that future studies examining genetics in a sex-specific framework be *a priori* based, with clearly defined context and adequately powered subgroups [Patsopoulos, et al, 2007]. In other words, without comparable data on both sexes in the same study, the very piece examining sex-specific variation is actually omitted from the puzzle [Bird and Rieker, 2008]. Further elaboration of physiological differences between the sexes may illuminate additional pathways affecting context-specific variation in gene expression, gene-by-environmental interaction, and patterns of morbidity and mortality [Luczak and Leinwand, 2009; Ordovas, 2007; Pilote, et al, 2007; Lawlor et al, 2001]. Due to the recent exponential identification of genes, we cite several reviews offering candidate genes for subsequent research.

THE LIPID TRANSPORT SYSTEM

Lipids

The structure and function of lipids is widely covered in current literature, well beyond the scope of this review. We shall only remind the reader of several relevant lipids and their functions. Fatty acids are a major source of fuel, structural components, and activation of transcription factors. They are packaged in triglycerides for transfer or storage in adipose tissue and muscle [Mittendorfer, 2005; Woollett, 2001]. Cholesterol, whose steroid nucleus is synthesized from fatty acid by-products, is a substantial component in growth and development. Cholesterol plays an integral part in: 1) cell membrane construction and dynamics [Hadley, 1985; Yeagle, 1990]; 2) development of brain, nervous system, and surfactant [Myant, 1991Woollett, 2001]; and 3) modulating functions of the oxytocin receptors [Gimpl et al, 2002], which, in turn, are found to express in a sex-specific manner in animals [Uhi-Bronner et al, 2005].

Water insoluble lipids are transported through the blood stream via a system of lipoprotein packages, classified by their relative load of triglycerides, phospholipids, cholesterol and apoproteins, the protein moieties of lipoproteins [Gropper, Smith and Groff,

2005]. Apoproteins serve a range of functions that include assembling the lipoproteins, acting as enzyme cofactors which facilitate lipid transfer between lipoproteins, to becoming ligands for lipoprotein receptors [Weiss, 1993; Mahley et al, 1984; Alaupovic, 1991; Ordovas and Corella, 2004]. The series of lipoprotein packages is primarily formed by bipolar phospholipids. Fats and cholesterol esters are sequestered in the hydrophobic core of fatty acid chains, while the hydrophilic phosphate heads form the outside package capable of being floated through the vascular system to the cells [Brown and Goldstein, 1986]. These lipoprotein entities are defined by their composition and density, which are affected by the differential lipid loads [Alaupovic, 1991]. The lipid transport system consists of three pathways; 1) a pathway specifically for the dietary source, 2) one for those endogenously produced, and 3) a reverse transport pathway by which the body removes excesses from the cells and tissues. Lipoproteins are cleared from plasma by both receptor-mediated and receptor-independent processes. Clearance rates through the former, but not the latter process are dependent upon plasma concentrations [Woollett, 2008].

Exogenous And Endogenous Pathways

Dietary fats and cholesterol are transported by the chylomicron (CM) lipoprotein formed in the small intestine. This lipoprotein moves the lipids through the lymphatic system and thoracic duct to the subclavian vein where it enters the bloodstream. Once CMs deliver their major load of diet-acquired energy to muscles and adipose tissue, their cholesterol-rich remnants are delivered to the liver. The CM is generally cleared from circulation within 12 hours [Voet and Voet, 1990], although females clear these faster than males [Knuth and Horowitz, 2006]. This male–female difference has been attributed different patterns of metabolically active adipose tissue [Couillard, et al, 1999; Horton et al, 2002].

The endogenous pathway originates in the liver, beginning the series of lipoproteins with very-low-density lipoprotein (VLDL), which delivers liver-synthesized triglycerides to the cells for energy. The low-density lipoprotein, (LDL), derived in part from remodeled VLDL remnants, primarily delivers cholesterol to the cells [Weiss, 1993]. During remodeling, the lipoprotein triglyercide percent is reduced from 52% in the VLDL to 9% in the LDL, increasing the percent of cholesterol from 22% in the VLDL to 47% in the LDL [Gropper, Smith and Groff, 2005]. In adults, approximately 60 % of circulating cholesterol is associated with LDL [Le and Walter, 2007]. Four classes of LDL have been identified [Gofman et al, 2007 for review], differing not only in their triglyceride percentage and dietary determinants, but also in their metabolic and pathogenic results [Krauss, 2001]. The apoproteins Bs, Cs and E (APOB, APOC1, 2, 3 and APOE) are the primary protein constituents of these lipoproteins carrying triglycerides and cholesterol to the cells.

Two notable enzymes affect this transport system: 1) hormone sensitive lipase (HSL)-- responsible for lypolysis in adipose tissue, thus releasing triglycerides to the liver for transport [Qi, et al, 2004]; 2) lipoprotein lipase (LPL), functioning in the opposite direction, i.e. adipocyte uptake of triglycerides from circulating lipoproteins [Votruba and Jensen, 2007]. HSL is located in adipose and steroidogenic tissue, regulating body fat and insulin secretion, while LPL is synthesized adipose, muscle, and other tissue involved with fatty acid metabolism. LPL activity is profoundly related to dietary intake [Karpe, et al, 1998]. Sex-specific variation in both enzymes is documented. Alcohol intake appears to influence one of HSLs genetic polymorphisms in a sex-specific manner [Qi, et al, 2004]. Greater LPL activity is reported in females than males and may be affected by the specific fat depot in which they reside, size of adipocytes, and macronutrient composition in the diet [Imbeault et la, 1999; Votruba and Jensen; 2007; Yost, et al, 1998]. The review reporting considerable heterogeneity in effects of LPL polymorphisms on HDL and TG levels did not address sex-specific variation [Sagoo et al 2008].

Reverse Transport System

The reverse transport system removes excess cholesterol from the cells through the activity of the high-density lipoprotein HDL, which carries 20-30% of circulating cholesterol [Le and Walter, 2007]. The primary apoprotein associated with HDL is A1, although apoprotein Cs and E are transferred from other lipoproteins to HDL during maturation [Weiss, 1993]. HDL is considered the most complex of the lipoproteins. Beyond its putative role of sequestering and transporting cholesterol and other detrimental products back to the liver for disposal, HDL delivers much of the cholesterol to the adrenals and ovary for steroidogenesis, inhibits endothelial inflammation and monocyte adehesion, and promotes production of endothelial nitric oxide (NO) and prostacyclins [Lewis and Rader, 2005]. It also appears to have an antioxidant quality by hydrolyzing damaged lipids (Brown, 2007.), an involvement with the acute-phase response and a role in complement regulation [Scanu and Edelstein, 2008].

HDL variation directly relating to sex hormones is documented, and studies indicate higher HDL levels associated with higher estrogen and lower HDL levels with higher testosterone [Khaw and Barrett-Conner]. This direct relationship is challenged; suggesting differences may not originate directly from physiological differences between the sexes, but reflect behavioral issues which attenuate the magnitude of variation [Davis et al, 1996]. Our recent research regarding genes, nutrition and serum lipids in two semi isolate populations indicate that HDL in males may be more directly vulnerable to total energy intake and nutrients, while female HDL highly correlated with central adipose tissue and related adipokines, but not with dietary variation. Similar findings are identified both in an indigenous population exhibiting one of the lowest serum lipid profiles worldwide and specifically in phytosterol intake in a population located in central Kansas, exhibiting average US lipid profiles [Mosher et al, 2005; Mosher et al, 2006; Mosher, Demarchi and Crawford, 2008]. See Figure 1: Lipid Transport

The protective effects of HDL levels do not appear consistent across populations, suggesting that gene and dietary factors not related to HDL quantity, but related to quality of its protective anti-inflammatory and antioxidant properties are also involve (Barter et al, 2003). For example, one of HDL's associated enzymes is paraoxonase (PON1), believed to prevent LDL and HDL oxidation [Rozek, et al., 2005]. PON1 activity is higher in females than in males [Kleemola et al, 2002] and recently demonstrated to have sex-specific genetic effects in a large familial-based study of 42 extended families of Mexican Americans [Winnier et al, 2007]. Further research suggests that variation in activity associated with its genetic polymorphisms is not consistent among populations [Senti, et al., 2002; Brophy, et al,

2001; Rozek, et al, 2005]. This variation is PON1 activity is independent of genotype, and therefore may be related to nutritional factors among the populations [Durrington et al, 2001]. PON1 activity showed sex specific responses to high-fat diets in animals [Thomas-Moya, et al, 2007] and dietary modifications in human females [Rantala, et al, 2002]. No study yet puts sex, genes and diet for a comprehensive look at PON1.

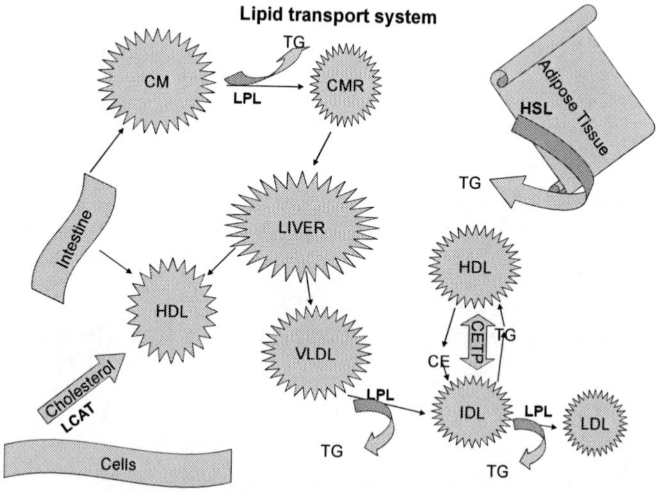

Figure 1: The lipid transport system- Chylomicrons (CM and their remnants (CMR) transport dietary fats from intestines to cells and liver. Very low density lipoprotein (VLDL) takes endogenous lipids from liver to cells. As triglycerides (TG) are downloaded from VLDL, lipoprotein remodeling results in intermediate density lipoprotein (IDL), then low density lipoprotein (LDL) which delivers cholesterol to cells. Lipoprotein lipase (LPL) releases triglycerides (TG) from lipoproteins and hormone sensitive lipase (HSL) releases TG from adipose tissue. The reverse transport takes lipids released from tissues by lecithin cholesterol acyl transferase (LCAT) and lipids released from other lipoproteins by cholesterol ester transfer protein (CETP) to gonads for hormone construction and to the liver for disposal. (Adapted from Gropper, Smith and Groff, 2005).

Several candidate genes involved in the remodeling of HDL have been examined for dietary effects, with inconsistent results. They are cholesterol ester transfer protein (CETP), involved in the exchange of lipids between lipoproteins, and lecithin cholesterol acyl transferase (LCAT), activated by APOA1 to facilitate cholesterol uptake from the cells and mature the HDL [Ye and Kwiterovich, 2000; Scanu and Edelstein, 2008]. Genes for both proteins are located on chromosome 16q in an area linked to QTL-by-sex interaction affecting HDL variation [Mosher, et al, 2005]. A family-derived haplotype in the CETP gene is also associated with lipid variation in males (Bauerfeind, et al, 2002). Additional key players are the enzyme hepatic lipase (HL) and its gene, LIPC. The HL enzyme is reported to be twice as high in males as in females, and females show a reduction of HL activity during the luteal phase of their menstrual cycle [Carr, et al, 2001]. Gene-by-diet interactions have been reported, yet there are no combined study of sex–specific dietary variation [Deeb et al, 2003]. Evidence of ethnic [Carr, et al, 2004], and dietary [Ordovas et al, 2002], but not sex effects [Isaacs et al, 2004], have been shown in the LIPC promoter region known as -514(C/T). An extensive review of additional genes involved in the regulation of cholesterol homeostasis is found in Martini and Pallottini [2007]. While this article does not address sex-specific effects, it does offer an excellent listing of potential candidate genes for future studies.

Sexual Dimorphism in Serum Lipids

A metabolic profile of lipids involves determining the major lipoprotein distribution. It may be extended to include lipoprotein subclasses, giving a more precise in examination of a disturbance in lipid metabolism [Gofman et al, 2007]. Gofman et al, report little sexual dimorphism is noted in the four LDL classes before the age of 15, with males exhibiting higher LDL levels until midlife, a point at which LDL in females may surpass male levels. HDL trends were not parallel to those of LDL, despite some age and sex differences. After examining the interclass relationships of LDL and HDL, these authors hypothesize that metabolic factors controlling lipoprotein trends may be different for LDL and HDL. The universality of these trends has not been fully explored, and may not be consistent with these reported trends which were determined solely on an American population consuming the Western diet [Gofman, et al, 2007].

Although some studies fail to report sexual dimorphism in lipid profiles until puberty [Sneider et al, 1997], those studies which describe differences beginning with the neonate consistently note female lipids to be higher than males [Bansal, et al, 2005; Carlson and Hardell, 1977; Pac-Kozuchowska, 2007]. They are explained by the additive estrogen levels produced by both maternal and fetal glands. Specifically, females are shown to have lower total cholesterol (TC) to HDL ratio than males [Nelson et al., 2007], a protective profile similar to one frequently observed in adult females profiles. Dyslipidemias in adolescence and adulthood may be affected by disproportionate growth patterns in response to nutritional deficits during critical developmental stages *in utero* [Barker, 1995; Godfrey, 2002 review]. Several studies, including those involving populations in the Philippines and Hong Kong, offered additional insight, and supported the hypothesis that male offspring appear to be more vulnerable to persistent effects on lipid metabolism associated with maternal nutrition and lower birth weight [Kuzawa and Adair, 2003; Lawler, et al, 2006]. These findings are consistent with Barker's fetal origin of disease hypothesis and possibly relate to the male's greater demand for energy to meet their more rapid growth *in utero* [Skidmore et al, 2004; Kuzawa and Adair, 2004]. Interestingly, a study of Chinese reported that improved nutrition which stimulates higher sex-hormones at puberty appears to be ultimately detrimental to males by producing atherogenic profiles and greater body fat, but did not affect females negatively [Schooling et al, 2007]. A systematic review of research examining the relationship of early nutritional stress on adolescent and adult lipids, reports inconsistent findings to support the relationship of fetal nutrition to total cholesterol, but this review did not examine the data from a sex-specific perspective [Owen et al, 2003].

Origins of Sexual Dimorphism in Serum Lipids

The current literature regarding causal relationships for set point or time of onset for sexual dimorphism in serum lipid profiles is sparse. Fetal programming results from a complex interaction of genetic and epigenetic factors, including the combination of parental genotypes and their imprinting, which involves expression of genes based upon parent of origin. This genetic conflict hypothesis suggests that paternal genes influence nutrient acquisition, thus encouraging growth. Maternal genes, on the other hand, are more conservative, both protecting the mother's resources while supporting fetal growth. All of these factors ultimately interact to influence both placental and fetal development [Myatt, 2006: Reik et al, 2003; Gallou-Kabani and Junien, 2005]. Further influencing offspring phenotype are factors such as grandmother's nutritional experience creating epigenetic changes, along with the maternal physiological response to pregnancy and ongoing nutritional status, influencing placental development and its capacity for nutrient transfer and ultimately fetal growth [Godfey, 2002; Jansson and Powell, 2007; Fowden et al., 2006; Woollett, 1995]. The timing of environmental insults is critical on placental or fetal development [Barker, 1995; Myatt, 2006], creating altered programming with life-long consequences [Nijland et al, 2008; Gilbert and Nijland, 2008]. The placenta is primary determinant of nutritional fetal support, responsive to both maternal and fetal signaling through glucose transporters (GLUT). Both nutritional factors and hormones such as growth hormone, glucocorticoids and leptin influence the transport system [Myatt, 2006; Fowden et al, 2006]. This communication between maternal and fetal systems may, in fact, represent a coadaptation, which some interpret as more influential on genetic imprinting [Wolf and Hager. 2006]. Thus, the resulting offspring phenotype may represent an adaptive response to maternal and fetal genetics and their intrauterine signals, with a subsequent developmental path adjusted to the environmental circumstances [Jansson and Powell, 2007].

Fetal triglyceride and cholesterol originate from both exogenous sources of maternal circulatory lipoproteins and endogenous synthesis. As the primary source of energy in fetal tissue is glucose oxidation, fatty acids are used for structural components or stored for energy at times of nutritional stress [Woollett, 2001]. Estrogen appears to regulate LDL receptors, as well as enhance uterine-placental blood flow and thus nutrient uptake [Pepe and Albrecht, 1995]. Early development of these LDL receptors is vital for fetal survival [Herz and Farese, 1999]. Fetal cholesterol synthesis, once begun, occurs at a much higher rate in the fetus than in the adult [Rainey et al 2002]. In fact, these higher rates continue in humans throughout the pregnancy, and do not decrease toward the end of gestation, contrary to other species [Woollett, 2008].

Postnatal cord blood is one manner by which lipid transport between the maternal and fetal circulation is assessed, with implications reaching into adulthood [Kelishadi et al 200; Bansal et al, 2005]. Cord lipoproteins correlate with cord levels of adipokines, leptin and adiponectin, but not birth weight [Lindsay et al, 2003]. Bansal et al. showed a strong inverse correlation of adiponectin with LDL levels, but not with HDL. Both findings were independent of maternal ethnicity and in contrast to the correlation between HDL and adiponectin found in adult studies [Bansal et al, 2006]. Cord blood levels of adiponectin are two to three times higher than found in adults, with fetal adiponectin located in a variety of fetal cells beyond the expected adipose and placental tissue. These findings suggest novel, yet unexplained action of adiponectin *in utero* [Corbetta, et al, 2005]. Fetal leptin cord blood levels are correlated with birth weight, are higher than their mothers levels, and show a decided sex-specific difference, not correlated with maternal levels. Female levels are higher than males [Tome et al, 1997; Schubring et al, 2006]. Leptin appears to have multiple roles during reproduction, as suggested by the variety of fetal tissues expressing leptin receptors.

Explanatory mechanisms are yet to be fully identified, but animal studies suggest fetal bone remodeling, promotion of hematopoiesis and lymphopoiesis, pulmonary development, and affecting intestinal mucosa maturation [Henson and Castracane, 2006; Alexe, et al, 2006]. Leptin is instrumental in the transitional time directly after birth, by regulating the uncoupling protein 1 (UCP1) involved in heat production of brown adipose tissue (BAT) [Alexe et al, 2006 for review].

Neonate variation in significant apoproteins and lipoprotein levels are also affected by maternal nutritional status. A comparison of Iranian mothers of varying preconception weights found an association in the cord levels of APOA in underweight mothers, and APOB levels associated with overweight mothers. Babies large for gestational age (LGA) also exhibited statistically higher LDL but lower HDL [Kalishadi et al, 2007], a study that did not determine sex effects. Additional factors influencing cord blood lipid profiles are reviewed in Bansal et al, [2005]. Neonate cholesterol levels range from 50-100mg/dl, in an equal balance of HDL and LDL. These levels double or triple within the first six months, with much of the increase expressed in LDL-- the primary lipoprotein to deliver cholesterol to the cells [Innis and Hamilton, 1992; Sneider et al, 2003]. Serum lipids are correlated with IGF-1 (growth factor) and the hormones leptin and adiponectin, released by the placenta. Leptin metabolism deregulation is indicated in the pathogenesis gestational diabetes [Lappas et al., 2005]. And, disruption of these hormone-lipid associations in offspring whose mothers have Type1 diabetes, show a sex-specific pattern, with males at jeopardy for long term effects [Nelson, et al, 2007]. Further review of nutritional affects on the development of gene-by-hormone receptors interaction, (ie. thyroid and glucocorticoid hormones),-tangentially related to growth and development, energy and metabolism and body composition-- is available in Dauncey et al [2001]. Research examining early programming and set points for these adipokines and lipoproteins may identify further causal pathways of lipid control.

Body Composition and Serum Lipids

Sexual dimorphism in body composition and fat patterning has been extensively studied, with most studies concentrating on the relationship between regional fat patterns and serum lipids [Despres, et al, 1990]. Increased understanding of sex-specific variation in muscle tissue, uncoupling proteins, substrate preference and their inter-relationship to problems such as obesity and Type 2 diabetes now offers a more complex picture of the relationship between body composition and serum lipids.

Lean Tissue

The development of body composition is influenced directly by sex hormones, which in turn indirectly influence the cascade of metabolically active signals mediating energy homeostasis, growth and development, the immune system and inflammatory processes. Due to testosterone males are predominately larger than females, with a greater proportion of bone mineral and lean muscle mass located especially in the upper body, while females exhibit a greater percentage of body fat due to estrogen [Nindl, et al., 2002; Wells, 2007]. As muscle is an energy-expensive tissue, males also maintain a higher basal metabolism rate [Wizemann and Pardue, 2001].

Human skeletal muscle is divided into three categories, a slow twitch (ST) or Type I and two fast twitch (FTa and FTb) or Type II [Simoneau and Bouchard, 1995], FTa has hybrid characteristics found in ST and FTb. ST muscle fibers, used for sustained activity, show higher levels of lipids and the mitochondria in which fatty acid β-oxidation occurs. FTb are considered glycolytic, with higher glycogen content. FTa fibers appear to have both lipid oxidation and glycolitic capabilities. Studies of the vastus lateralis muscle in sedentary individuals showed males had lower capacity for lipid oxidation than females, while females showed a reduced use of glycogen [Ettinger, 1999]. These findings are not consistent when other muscle groups are compared, although sex-specific ratios of the different muscle types support the hypothesis that females have more Type I fibers [Chorneyko and Bourgeois, 1999] and preferentially utilize β-oxidation to obtain energy [Wizemann and Pardue,2001]. Moreover, during times of increased energy expenditure, estrogen upregulates fat oxidation in females, while males upregulate use of carbohydrate and protein as their substrates of choice [Power and Schulkin, 2008]. Further indication of sex-specific variation was identified using oligonucleotide microarrays of skeletal tissue. Unexpectedly, males had higher expression of genes for mitochondrial proteins along with greater translation initiation capability, which the authors interpreted as supporting a greater rate of protein synthesis per muscle fiber in males [Welle et al, 2008]. Nutritional implications of these differences for serum lipid variation are not fully explored.

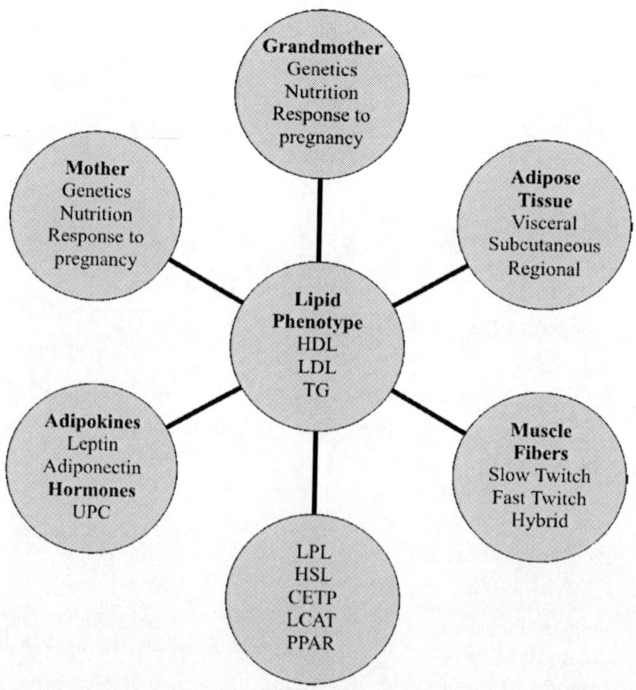

Figure 2: Aspects of sexual dimorphism affecting lipid phenotypes of HDL-high-density lipoprotein, LDL-low density lipoprotein, TG-triglyceride. Factors include genetics, epigenetics, body composition and its variation, adipokines, muscle fibers, uncoupling proteins (UCP), enzymes lipoprotein lipase (LPL), hormone sensitive lipase (HSL), cholesterol ester transfer protein (CETP), lecithin cholesterol acyl transferase (LCAT), and peroxisome proliferator activated receptors (PPAR).

ADIPOSE TISSUE

Once thought to be merely a storage depot for triglycerides, adipose tissue, is now recognized to be an active participant in the regulation of energy homeostasis. It performs as an endocrine gland, i.e. releasing bioactive peptides affecting a range of energy related functions. These peptides, or adipokines, include leptin, adiponectin, PPAR-γ, LPL, CETP, uncoupling proteins, and steroid hormones. They form a multi-organ communication network regulating such issues as food intake, energy balance, insulin sensitivity, lipid metabolism, and inflammation, [Yu and Ginsberg, 2005; Ronti et al, 2006; Meier and Gressner, 2004]. Additionally, there are two forms of adipose tissue, with opposing functions: 1) white adipose tissue (WAT), the tissue with which we are most familiar, channels lipids toward energy storage; and 2) brown adipose tissue (BAT), functions in an adaptive or non-shivering thermogenesis, using lipid oxidation to release heat [Klaus and Keijer, 2004]. Despite traditional thinking that these two cells arise may from the same preadipocytes, the mechanisms underlying fat cell differentiation during development are poorly understood and may, in fact, point to different origins [Gaetani, 2008].

BROWN ADIPOSE TISSUE AND UNCOUPLING PROTEINS

In humans, BAT, develops early *in utero*, specifically in interscapular, pericardial and perirenal regions. Innervated by the sympathetic nervous system, BAT is also highly vascular, and contains many mitochondria [Hansen and Kristiansen 2006]. Cells of both BAT and WAT may be found interspersed in the same fat depots, with the percentage of BAT reducing substantially during the first year of life. Originally believed to disappear by adulthood, BAT has been documented in older adults living in northern climates. [Hassi, 1977; Leppaluoto and Hassi, 1989]. Heat is generated from BAT as a result of uncoupling protein 1 (UCP1), an inner mitochondrial membrane transporter that uncouples the oxidation of fuel substrates from adenosine triphosphate (ATP) production, thus dissipating potential energy as heat [Argyropoulos and Harper, 2002]. Greater quantities of UCP-1 have also been associated with visceral adipose depots in adults [Hansen and Kristiansen, 2006].

Additional uncoupling proteins have been identified. UCP2 is found in skeletal muscle, white adipose tissue, pancreatic islets and the central nervous system and UCP3 is predominantly expressed in skeletal muscle [Hamada et al, 2008]. Nutritional studies suggest a role of these two in substrate fuel utilization in muscle (Argyropoulous and Harper, 2002). Polymorphisms in UCP-1 are associated with variation in LDL, HDL and atherogenic index [Oh et al, 2004], and UCP-2 affects variation in LDL particle size [Hamada et al, 2008], and in hypertension [Kotani et al, 2007]. Sex differences in uncoupling protein action have been associated in diet, weight, and cold-induced studies on animals [Rodriguez and Palou, 2004; Valle et al, 2008]. Recent connections of BAT and uncoupling proteins with diabetes, obesity and serum lipid variation, are now stimulating renewed interest in this area.

White Adipose Tissue and Adipokines

White adipose tissue (WAT) differs from BAT both in predominant anatomical location and metabolic function. Beyond its putative role of energy storage, WAT secretes at least 26 adipokines, many of which influence lipid metabolism and insulin resistance. Sex steroid hormones are directly responsible for much of the difference in body composition, and patterning [Wells, 2007]. Human sexual dimorphism is widely documented in variation of body composition and fat patterning, and more interestingly, in fat metabolism, gene expression in adipose tissue and even the energy content of weight change [Blaak, 2001; Votruba and Jensen, 2007; Klaus and Keijer, 2004; Pietrobelli et al, 2002] A recent review supports the consistent finding across populations -- that females possess greater amounts of adipose stores than males, a phenomenon present at birth [Power and Schulkin, 2008; Wells, 2007]. Ethnic comparisons have shown the relative body mass index to percent body fat and fat patterning is more consistent across populations in males than in females [Fernandez et al, 2003; Wang et al, 1994; Gallagher et al, 1996].

Sex differences in body composition begin after age six, when body fat content increases in females, while lean mass increases in males. At puberty, the variation in fat patterning becomes more pronounced and by adulthood, distinct patterns are observed in fat distribution. In males fat deposits accumulate primarily on the trunk and abdomen as visceral fat in the omentum and mesentery, while females deposit fat on the buttocks, thighs and in subcutaneous abdominal regions [Klaus and Keijer, 2004]. The sex differences of abdominal fat depot (males in visceral, females in subcutaneous) have been substantiated by MRI, with body composition remaining more consistent in females than males with age [Kuk et al, (2005].

Dimorphic fat patterning is attributed to sex hormones. While receptors to the androgen and estrogen hormones are present in both sexes, the hormone levels regulate sex-hormone binding globulins and availability of free hormones to target tissues, thus regulating fat accumulation patterns [Federman, 2006]. Testosterone affects muscle development, inhibits LPL activity, decreases TG accumulation, and increases lypolysis. In contrast, estrogen, converted from testosterone by aromatase [Federman, 2006], affects subcutaneous fat deposition, food intake and energy expenditure, as well as enhancing the proliferation of preadipocytes in both sexes. The subcutaneous fat in females appears to have greater sensitivity to estrogen's effect of decreasing lipolysis and proliferation of preadipocytes [Power and Schulkin, 2008]. The regional differences in fat patterning have distinct implications for metabolism and substrate use. Fatty acid uptake in females is higher in the thigh, and abdominal subcutaneous fat. In males, not only is fatty acid uptake greater in visceral fat of the abdomen, the rate of turnover is also greater [Williams, 2004]. Substrate use during times of increased energy expenditure also differs. Here, females again show preference of fats for fuels. as estrogen upregulates fat oxidation. This increased utilization of fat by females does not appear to be related to amount of fat composition of the body [Norgan 1997]. Males, on the other hand, upregulate use of carbohydrates and protein for their substrates of choice [Power and Schulkin, 2008]. Interestingly, basal fat oxidation may actually be less in females than in males after adjusting for fat free mass [Blaak, 2001], thus allowing time for fat storage.

The metabolic implications for visceral fat are also associated with greater risk of dyslipidemias and problems of glucose metabolism. Ethnic variation in susceptibility to accumulation of visceral fat and specific health problems is documented, however [Cossrow and Falkner, 2004]. Additionally results of *in vitro* studies of human adipose tissue suggest a gender-specific variation in the ratio of adrenoreceptor subtypes and susceptibility to catecholamines which effect lypolysis [Williams, 2004, for discussion]. After menopause, such sex-specific differences decrease substantially [Wizemann and Perdue, 2001], with increase central fat in females [Williams, 2004]. Animal studies addressing energy homeostasis suggest that substrate preference is manifested by the arcuate nucleus in the brain, describing a neurological pathway involving α-melanocyte stimulating hormone (α-MSH) and proopiomelanocorticotropin (POMC) melanocyte whereby females are more sensitive to leptin signals and males to insulin signals [Woods, et al, 2003].

Table 1. Comparison of adipokines leptin and adiponectin, both synthesized in adipose tissue.

Leptin	Adiponectin
Dimorphic from birth	No dimorphism at birth
Signals Satiety	Dimorphic in adulthood
Stimulates fatty acid oxidation in muscles	Stimulates glucose uptake and utilization
Inhibits TG accumulation in liver	Increases insulin sensitivity
Normal levels a prerequisite for onset of puberty reproductive function	Inverse correlation with TG Positive correlation with HDL and LPL
Increased by estrogen	Increased by estrogen
Suppressed by testosterone	Suppressed by testosterone

ADIPOKINES

The endocrine function of adipose tissue is manifested through the release of adipokines, bioactive protein communicators [see review Ronti et al, 2006]. Sexual dimorphism is substantially documented in several adipokines, including leptin and adiponectin, even after adjustment for percentages of body fat [Guerra et al, 2008]. Their importance in fetal development has been previously detailed in this article. Leptin, is highly expressed in subcutaneous WAT and possibly BAT [Margetic et al, 2002], while adiponectin release is associated consistently with visceral fat depots [Klaus and Keijer, 2004]. Plasma levels of adiponectin are negatively associated with increased body fat mass and insulin resistance [Ong, et al, 2006]. Two additional adipokines inhibit adiponectin. They are interleukin-6 (IL6) which increases hepatic *de novo* synthesis of fatty acids and cholesterol and tumor necrosis factor (TNF), which stimulates release of free fatty acids from adipose tissue [Ronti, et al, 2006]. Estrogen increases levels of both leptin and adiponectin, thus enhancing their levels during reproduction [Mitchell, et al., 2005]. Testosterone suppresses adiponectin [Bottner et al, 2004] and leptin levels [Lukkaa et al, 1998], suggesting one manner by which male may be more vulnerable to disorders of insulin and lipid metabolism.

Leptin

Leptin plays a substantial role in energy homeostasis, reducing food intake and stimulating energy expenditure [Parcchini et al, 2005]. It serves to improve insulin sensitivity peripherally through its actions of reducing intracellular lipid levels in skeletal muscle and liver and decreasing insulin production in pancreatic β cells, as well as antagonizing insulin action [Mitchell et al, 2005]. Additionally, it is thought to increase energy expenditure through its involvement with elevated sympathetic activity and UCP activity [Cortright, 1999]. From birth females have higher levels of leptin than males due to the elevating effects of estrogen and adipose tissue [Alexe et al, 2006], yet females show a greater lowering of leptin during aerobic training than males. This suggests a mechanism of energy conservation for the female [Cortright, 1999; Margetic, et al 2002, review]. The greater responsiveness of females to leptin is believed to be secondary to the blunting role estrogen plays on insulin's central effects. Males, due to their greater percentage of visceral than central subcutaneous fat, are more sensitive to insulin signals. Males are also more susceptible to the detrimental effects of increased visceral tissue, as their rates of lipolysis and lipogenesis are greater than in females [Power and Schulkin, 2008]. Testosterone levels are inversely correlated to leptin levels and the expression of specific leptin receptors in skeletal muscle [Welle et al, 2008], although no correlation was noted between serum levels and leptin receptors in either males or females [Guerra et al., 2008]. Through its affects on the hypothalamic-pituitary-gonadal axes, leptin plays a vital role in fertility and pregnancy [Meier and Gressner, 2004], and this reproductive connection may explain why female levels are inherently higher.

Adiponectin

Adiponectin, primarily known for its antiatherogenic properties shows a positive correlation with HDL levels in both males and females, and a negatively association with triglyderide levels and insulin resistance [Ronti, et al., 2006]. Insulin increases adiponectin synthesis in WAT, which in turn enhances insulin sensitivity through such roles as suppressing hepatic glucose production and lipid synthesis, reducing blood glucose and free fatty acid concentrations, and increasing gene expression of UPC2 in muscle. Fatty acid oxidation in both muscle and liver is increased [Meier and Gressner, 2004; Yamauchi et al, 2002; Matsubara et al, 2002]. Adiponectin synthesis and secretion are affected by the size of adipocytes, with increases in secretion associated with small adipocytes, and decreases seen with adipocyte hypertrophy [Meier and Gressner, 2004]. In adults, adiponectin levels are negatively associated with the visceral adipose tissue and negatively associated with leptin levels in females [Matsubara et al, 2002]. Adult levels are dimorphic, a difference from the higher newborns levels previously mentioned, which are not sexually dimorphic. Moreover the neonate adiponectin levels are independent of birth weight [Lindsay, et al, 2003].

PPAR

Interrelated with both leptin and adiponectin are the peroxisome proliferator-actived receptors, PPARα and PPARγ. and PPARβ/δ. Members of the nuclear hormone receptor super family, they serve as ligand-activated transcription factors which regulate both glucose and lipid metabolism. PPARγ is highly expressed in adipose tissue, where it regulates adipocytes differentiation adipocytes and fat metabolism. It is also located in muscle and endothelial tissue, influencing insulin sensitivity [Lovegrove and Gitau, 2008; Cecil et al, 2006; Memisoglu et al, 2003; Paracchini et al, 2005]. Fatty acids and eicosanoid metabolites are among the ligands and activators of these receptors [Nakamura et al, 2004; Barbier et al, 2002]. PPARs play a central role in fatty acid metabolism, and influence the reverse transport system through HDL by cholesterol efflux from macrophages and bile acid synthesis. Additionally, they increase adiponectin receptor expression [Tsuchid et al, 2005], accentuating the protective role of HDL, through regulation of cellular adhesion to endothelial cells and repression of thrombin-induced vasoconstrictors [Barbier et al, 2002]. *In utero*, PPARs express early, regulating placental and fetal development. Research suggests that these receptors play a distinct role in fetal adaptation to maternal diet and ultimate development of lipid metabolism, thus presenting an epigenetic mechanism by which fetal origin of lipid metabolism and disease outcome manifests [Rees, et al, 2007]. Animal studies examining PPARs and lipid homeostasis in the heart itself, report sex based differences [Luczak and Leinwand, 2009 –review]. Early studies show conflicting evidence for gene-by-diet interaction, but indicate some relationship to BMI and HDL variation [Lovegrove and Gitau, 2007; Ordovas and Corella, 2004]. Genotype-by-sex variation has been identified with longevity studies [Barbari et al, 2004] and in association with TG levels, but without a dietary component in the study [Khan et al, 2004]. The extensive relationships identified for PPARs, lipids, diet, and cardiac muscle are not fully documented, yet strongly suggest a sex-specific models for future research.

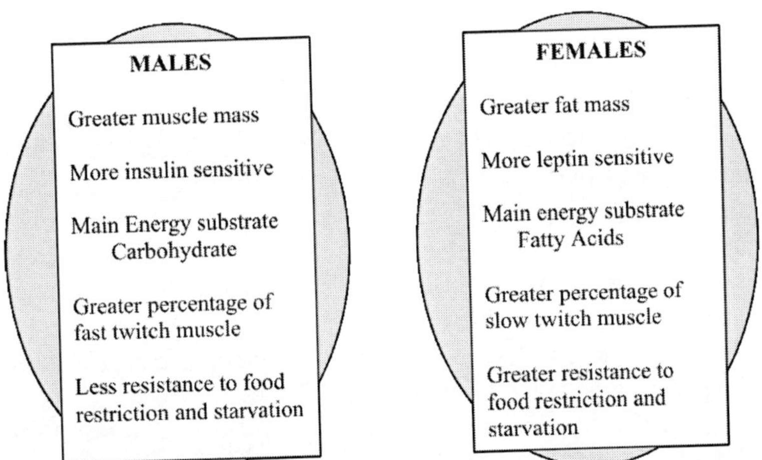

Figure 3: Sex-specific variation of body composition and related factors in untrained individuals.

Macronutrients and Energy

From an evolutionary perspective, given that the caloric density of fats is double that of both protein and carbohydrate, the apparent preference for greater fat storage and utilization in females can be seen as a reproductive advantage, especially during pregnancy and lactation [Wells, 2007]. Their additional advantage of the smaller body size, less muscle mass and lower basal metabolism which enhances energy storage all contribute to adaptations and differential survival of females during times of nutritional stress [Wizemann and Pardue, 2001; Cortright, 1999]. Deciphering the studies concerning sex-specific macronutrient intake and metabolism is extraordinarily complex due to the heterogeneity of methodologies and lack of standardization defining participant physiology. Variations involve fuels at rest versus during exercise, trained versus untrained, under hypoxic stress, and timing of female menstrual cycle. Estrogen alone promotes insulin sensitivity and glucose uptake in skeletal muscle and adipose tissue, while progesterone alone decreases insulin effects on these tissues. Current thought suggests that the ratio between these two hormones (estrogen and progesterone) may be a factor affecting variation in females' response to carbohydrate intake, especially under resting conditions [Ruby, 1999; see review]. The liver, skeletal muscle and central nervous system are the primary sites for glucose uptake in both males and females, with females having added demands in both uterine and placental tissues. Sex-specific variation in cerebral tissue glucose metabolism shows females to have 19 % higher rates than males, most likely associated with higher estrogen levels [Baxter, et al, 1987; Shi and Simpkins 1997]. As stated previously, during exercise, studies females oxidize less carbohydrate, and these studies suggest that females exhibit a lower glucose rate of appearance denoting less glucose production by the liver [Tarnopolsky 2003]. Carbohydrate loading, commonly used by athletes prior to an event, is now demonstrated to be effective for increasing muscle glycogen stores primarily in males, with females showing only slight increases in skeletal glucose during the female luteal phase. No post exercise glycogen resynthesis variation is reported between sexes [Ruby, 1999; Tarnopolsky, 2003]. Glucose challenges suppress nonesterfied fatty acid levels in females to a greater extent than in males. These differences have been replicated in several ethnic groups [McKeigue, et al, 1993].

Approximately three to six percent of total energy cost during extensive exercise is attributed to amino acid oxidation, and seven of the amino acids are known to be oxidized by human muscle [Phillips, 1999].. Sex-specific variation of specific oxidation in two of those amino acids, leucine and lysine, have been reported [Lamont, 2003]. Research in this area is scarce, except in studies involving athletic endurance [Phillips, 1999]. Protein use varies between the sexes, as seen in exercise studies and starvation studies. Both indicate that males catabolize more protein than do females. Although females metabolize less protein for energy, they may be more prone to inadequate protein intake and negative nitrogen balance, especially when facing dietary restrictions for esthetics or weight control coupled with increase in exercise. As in carbohydrate metabolism, protein catabolism in females may be related to the progesterone/estrogen ratio [Lamont et al, 2003; Phillips, 1999]. Higher protein diets are reported to lower serum triglycerides, but these effects may be secondary to the fat and carbohydrate content in the diet [Hu, 2005; Clifton and Keogh, 2007]. A randomized trial comparing diets reported a high protein diet lowered both LDL and HDL in both sexes [Appel, et al, 2005].

Sexual dimorphism in fat metabolism has been referenced throughout this review. To review, females preferentially store more body fat than males, and utilize fat as a primary energy substrate. Additionally, they show greater flexibility and control over free fatty acid homeostasis and exhibit a higher fatty acid release in relationship to their lower energy requirements [Power and Schulkin, 2008; Mittendorfer, 2005]. Much of this activity is attributed to estrogen and leptin [Power and Schulkin, 2008]. Differential sex-specific sensitivity to insulin's inhibiting effects on lypolysis and an adrenal medullary response to exercise also influence lipid homeostasis [Mittenddorfer, 2005].

Beyond differences in substrate metabolism, recent research offers novel considerations, suggesting genetic regulation of energy intake and even macronutrient preference. Linkage studies identify ethnic differences in quantitative trait loci (QTL) for dietary energy and individual macronutrient intake [Collaku et al, 2004] and distinct sex-specific linkage signals at a (QTL) influencing fasting insulin variation in females [North et al, 2007]. The complexity found in the new field of Nutrigenomics, understanding the relationship of nutritional effects on genotype to phenotype development over an entire life cycle, is daunting. Generational and epigenetic factors, nutritional effects on gene expression in growth and development, context specific metabolic demands and fluctuating nutritional requirements all represent pieces of the total puzzle. To ignore sex-differences when studying these relationships is no longer an option.

CONCLUSION

This review documents the importance of incorporating an environmental component (sex-specific variation) when constructing the architecture of complex traits such as lipid levels of the blood. Human sexual dimorphism associated with nutritional priorities involving fats and cholesterol is primarily under genetic control, but becomes attuned to environmental fluctuations *in utero*, and is intricately tied to reproductive requirements of the species. It is this interaction which affects the development and fluctuation of lipid phenotypes throughout the life cycle. Sexual variation in body composition, type of muscle content, metabolic active adipose tissue and adipokines, impact lipid transport, and result in the inconsistency reported by many gene and diet studies. Unraveling the relationship of genes and nutritional interactions must consider the complexities involved in the physiology of lipids as well as their evolutionary role.

REFERENCES

[1] Adair, LS; Prentice AM. A critical evaluation of the fetal origins hypothesis and its implications for developing countries. *J Nutr.*, 2004, 134(1), 191-3.

[2] Alaupovic, P. Apolipoprotein composition as the basis for classifying plasma lipoproteins. Characterization of ApoA- and ApoB-containing lipoprotein families. *Prog Lipid Res.,* 1991, 30(2-3), 105-38.

[3] Alexe, DM; Syridou, G; Petridou, ET. Determinants of early life leptin levels and later life degenerative outcomes. *Clin Med Res.,* 2006, 4(4), 326-35.

[4] Appel, LJ; Sacks, FM; Carey, VJ; Obarzanek, E; Swain, JF; Miller, ER., 3rd; et al. Effects of protein, monounsaturated fat, and carbohydrate intake on blood pressure and serum lipids: results of the OmniHeart randomized trial. *Jama*, 2005, 294(19), 2455-64.
[5] Argyropoulos, G; Harper, ME. Uncoupling proteins and thermoregulation. *J Appl Physiol.,* 2002, 92(5), 2187-98.
[6] Bansal, N; Charlton-Menys, V; Pemberton, P; McElduff, P; Oldroyd, J; Vyas, A., et al. Adiponectin in umbilical cord blood is inversely related to low-density lipoprotein cholesterol but not ethnicity. *J Clin Endocrinol Metab.,* 2006, 91(6), 2244-9.
[7] Bansal, N; Cruickshank, JK; McElduff, P; Durrington, PN. Cord blood lipoproteins and prenatal influences. *Curr Opin Lipidol.,* 2005, 16(4), 400-8.
[8] Barbier, O; Pineda Torra, I; Duguay, Y; Blanquart, C; Fruchart, JC; Glineur, C; Staels, B. Pleiotropic actions of peroxisome proliferator-activated receptors in lipid metabolism and atherosclerosis. *Arterioscler Thromb Vasc Biol.,* 2002, 22, 717-726.
[9] Barbieri, M; Bonafe, M; Rizzo, MR; Ragno, E; Olivieri, F; Marchegiani, F., et al. Gender specific association of genetic variation in peroxisome proliferator-activated receptor (PPAR)gamma-2 with longevity. *Exp Gerontol.,* 2004, 39(7), 1095-100.
[10]Barker, DJ. Fetal origins of coronary heart disease. *Bmj.,* 1995, 311(6998), 171-4.
[11]Barter, P; Kastelein, J; Nunn, A; Hobbs, R. High density lipoproteins (HDLs) and atherosclerosis; the unanswered questions. *Atherosclerosis*, 2003, 168(2), 195-211.
[12]Bauerfeind, A; Knoblauch, H; Schuster, H; Luft, FC; Reich, JG. Single nucleotide polymorphism haplotypes in the cholesteryl-ester transfer protein (CETP) gene and lipid phenotypes. *Hum Hered,* 2002, 54(4), 166-73.
[13]Baxter, L; Mazziotta, JC; Phelps, ME; Selin, CE; Guze, BH; Fairbankes, L. Cerebral glucose metabolic rates in normal human females versus normal males. *Psychiatry Research*, 1987, 21, 237.
[14]Bird C. and Reiker, P. Gender and Health. Cambridge: *Cambridge University Press,* 2008.
[15]Blaak, E. Gender differences in fat metabolism. *Curr Opin Clin Nutr Metab Care,* 2001, 4(6), 499-502.
[16]Bottner, A; Kratzsch, J; Muller, G; Kapellen, TM; Bluher, S; Keller, E., et al. Gender differences of adiponectin levels develop during the progression of puberty and are related to serum androgen levels. *J Clin Endocrinol Metab,* 2004, 89(8), 4053-61.
[17]Braunstein, G. Testes. In: Greenspan, F; Baxter; JD; editor. Basic and Clinical Endocrinology. 4th ed. Nowalk: *Appleton & Lange,* 1994. p. 391-418.
[18]Brophy, VH; Jampsa, RL; Clendenning, JB; McKinstry, LA; Jarvik, GP; Furlong, CE. Effects of 5' regulatory-region polymorphisms on paraoxonase-gene (PON1) expression. *Am J Hum Genet.,* 2001, 68(6), 1428-36.
[19]Brown, MS; Goldstein, JL. A receptor-mediated pathway for cholesterol homeostasis. *Science,* 1986, 232(4746), 34-47.
[20]Brown, W. High-density lipoprotein and transport of cholesterol and triglyceride in blood. *Journal of Clinical Lipidology,* 2007, 1, 7-19.
[21]Carlson, LA; Hardell, LI. Sex differences in serum lipids and lipoproteins at birth. *Eur J Clin Invest,* 1977, 7(2), 133-5.
[22]Carr, MC; Brunzell, JD; Deeb, SS. Ethnic differences in hepatic lipase and HDL in Japanese, black, and white Americans: role of central obesity and LIPC polymorphisms. *J Lipid Res.,* 2004, 45(3), 466-73.

[23]Carr, MC; Hokanson, JE; Zambon, A; Deeb, SS; Barrett, PH; Purnell, JQ, et al. The contribution of intraabdominal fat to gender differences in hepatic lipase activity and low/high density lipoprotein heterogeneity. *J Clin Endocrinol Metab,* 2001, 86(6), 2831-7.

[24]Cecil, JE; Watt, P; Palmer, CN; Hetherington, M. Energy balance and food intake: the role of PPARgamma gene polymorphisms. *Physiol Behav,* 2006, 88(3), 227-33.

[25]Chorneyko, K. and Bourgeois, J. Gender differences in skeletal muscle histology and ultrastructure. In: Tarnopolsky M; editor. Gender differences in metabolism: practical and nutritional implications. Boca Raton: CRC Press; 1999. p. 37-59.

[26]Clifton, PM; Keogh, J. Metabolic effects of high-protein diets. *Curr Atheroscler Rep.,* 2007, 9(6), 472-8.

[27]Collaku, A; Rankinen, T; Rice, T; Leon, AS; Rao, DC; Skinner, JS., et al. A genome-wide linkage scan for dietary energy and nutrient intakes: the Health, Risk Factors, Exercise Training, and Genetics (HERITAGE) Family Study. *Am J Clin Nutr.,* 2004, 79(5), 881-6.

[28]Corbetta, S; Bulfamante, G; Cortelazzi, D; Barresi, V; Cetin, I; Mantovani, G., et al. Adiponectin expression in human fetal tissues during mid- and late gestation. *J Clin Endocrinol Metab,* 2005, 90(4), 2397-402.

[29]Corella, D; Ordovas, JM. Single nucleotide polymorphism that influcence lipid metabolism interaction with dietary factors. *Annu Rev Nutr.,* 2005, 25, 341-90.

[30]Cortright. Sex differencces in regulation of energy homeostasis, growth and body composition furing periods of energy imbalance: anaimal studies. In: Tarnopolsky M, editor. Gender differences in metabolism: practical and nutritional implications. Boca Raton: CRC Press, 1999. p. 201-247.

[31]Cossrow, N; Falkner, B. Race/ethnic issues in obesity and obesity-related comorbidities. *J Clin Endocrinol Metab,* 2004, 89(6), 2590-4.

[32]Couillard, C; Bergeron, N; Prud'homme, D; Bergeron, J; Tremblay, A; Bouchard, C; Despres, JP. Gender differences in postprandial lipemia: importance of visceral adipose tissue accumulation. *Arterioscler Thromb Vasc Biol.,* 1999, 19(24), 2448-2455.

[33]Dauncey, MJ; White, P; Burton, KA; Katsumata, M. Nutrition-hormone receptor-gene interactions: implications for development and disease. *Proc Nutr Soc.,* 2001, 60(1), 63-72.

[34]Davis, CE; Williams, DH; Oganov, RG; Tao, SC; Rywik, SL; Stein, Y., et al. Sex difference in high density lipoprotein cholesterol in six countries. *Am J Epidemiol.,* 1996, 143(11), 1100-6.

[35]Deeb, SS; Zambon, A; Carr, MC; Ayyobi, AF; Brunzell, JD. Hepatic lipase and dyslipidemia: interactions among genetic variants, obesity, gender, and diet. *J Lipid Res.,* 2003, 44(7), 1279-86.

[36]Despres, JP; Moorjani, S; Lupien, PJ; Tremblay, A; Nadeau, A; Bouchard, C. Regional distribution of body fat, plasma lipoproteins, and cardiovascular disease. *Arteriosclerosis,* 1990, 10(4), 497-511.

[37]Durrington, PN; Mackness, B; Mackness, MI. Paraoxonase and atherosclerosis. *Arterioscler Thromb Vasc Biol.,* 2001, 21(4), 473-80.

[38]Ernst, N; Fisher, M; Bowen, P; Schaefer, EJ; Levy, RI. Changes in plasma lipids and lipoproteins after a modified fat diet. *Lancet,* 1980, 2(8186), 111-3.

[39]Ettinger, S. Muscle symppthetic nerve activity durig exercise and influences of gender. In: Tarnopolsky M; editor. Gender differences in metabolism: principal and nutritional implications. Boca Raton: CRC Press, 1999.

[40]Federman, DD. The biology of human sex differences. *N Engl J Med.,* 2006, 354(14), 1507-14.

[41]Fernandez, JR; Heo, M; Heymsfield, SB; Pierson, RN; Jr., Pi-Sunyer FX, Wang ZM; et al. Is percentage body fat differentially related to body mass index in Hispanic Americans, African Americans, and European Americans? *Am J Clin Nutr.,* 2003, 77(1), 71-5.

[42]Fowden, AL, Ward, JW; Wooding, FP; Forhead, AJ; Constancia, M. Programming placental nutrient transport capacity. *J Physiol*, 2006, 572(Pt 1), 5-15.

[43]Frikke-Schmidt, R; Sing, CF; Nordestgaard, BG; Tybjaerg-Hansen, A. Gender- and age-specific contributions of additional DNA sequence variation in the 5' regulatory region of the APOE gene to prediction of measures of lipid metabolism. *Hum Genet*, 2004, 115(4), 331-45.

[44]Gaetani, S. A sideways glance: does the color matter? A revised model of the origin of white and brown fat cells. *Genes Nutr.,* 2008, 3(3-4), 99-100.

[45]Gallagher, D; Visser, M; Sepulveda, D; Pierson, RN; Harris, T; Heymsfield, SB. How useful is body mass index for comparison of body fatness across age, sex and ethnic groups? *American Journal of Clinical Nutrition,* 1996, 143(3), 228-239.

[46]Gallou-Kabani, C; Junien, C. Nutritional epigenomics of metabolic syndrome: new perspective against the epidemic. *Diabetes,* 2005, 54(7), 1899-906.

[47]Gilbert, JS; Nijland, MJ. Sex differences in the developmental origins of hypertension and cardiorenal disease. *Am J Physiol Regul Integr Comp Physiol,* 2008, 295(6), R1941-52.

[48]Gimpl, G; Wiegand, V; Burger, K; Fahrenholz, F. Cholesterol and steroid hormones: modulators of oxytocin receptor function. *Prog Brain Res.,* 2002, 139, 43-55.

[49]Ginsberg, YYaH. Adipocyte signaling and lipid homeostasis: Sequelae of insulin-resistant adipose tissue. *Circ Res.,* 2005, 96, 1042-1052.

[50]Godfrey, KM. The role of the placenta in fetal programming-a review. *Placenta,* 2002, 23 Suppl A, S20-7.

[51]Gofman, J; Delalla, O; Glazier, F; Freeman, NK; Lindgren, FT; Nichols, AV; Strisower, B; Tamplin, AR. The serum lipoprotein transport system in health, metabolic disorders, atherosclerosis and coronary heart disease. *Journal of Clinical Lipidology,* 2007, 1(2), 104-141.

[52]Goldfien, A. and Monroe, SE. Ovaries. In: Baxter FGaJ, editor. Basic and Clinical Endocrinology. 4th ed. Norwalk: *Appleton & Lange.,* 1994. p. 419-470.

[53]Greil, H. Patterns of sexual dimorphism from birth to senescence. *Coll Antropol,* 2006, 30(3), 637-41.

[54]Gropper, S; Smith, JL; Groff, JL. Advanced nutrition and human metabolism. Fourth ed. Belmont: *Thomson Wadsworth,* 2005.

[55]Guerra, B; Fuentes, T; Delgado-Guerra, S; Guadalupe-Grau, A; Olmedillas, H; Santana, A., et al. Gender dimorphism in skeletal muscle leptin receptors, serum leptin and insulin sensitivity. PLoS ONE 2008, 3(10), e3466.

[56]Hadley, N. The adaptive role of lipids in biological systems. New York: *John Wiley and Sons,* 1985.

[57]Hamada, T; Kotani, K; Fujiwara, S; Sano, Y; Domichi, M; Tsuzaki, K; Takahhashi, K; Sakane, N. The UCP2-866 A/A genotype is associated with low density lipoprotein particle sizes in the general population. *Med Sci Monit,* 2008, 14(3), CR107-111.

[58]Hansen, JaKK. Regulatory circuits controlling white versus brown adipocyte differentiation. *Biochem J.* 2006, 398, 153-168.

[59]Hassi, J. The brown adipose tissue in man: structural and functional aspects in relation to age. Oulu: *University of Oulu,* 1977.

[60]Henson, MC, Castracane, VD. Leptin in pregnancy: an update. *Biol Reprod.,* 2006, 74(2), 218-29.

[61]Herz, J, Farese, RV., Jr. The LDL receptor gene family, apolipoprotein B and cholesterol in embryonic development. *J Nutr.,* 1999, 129(2S Suppl), 473S-475S.

[62]Horton, TJ; Commerford, SR; Pagliassotti, MJ; Bessesen, DH. Postprandial leg uptake of triglyceride is greater in women than in men. *Am J Physiol Endocrinol Metab.,* 2002, 283(6), E1192-202.

[63]Hu, F. Protein, body weight, and cardiovascular health. *Am J Clin Nutr.,* 2005, 82, (suppl), 242S-247S.

[64]Hubacek, J; Lanska, V; Skodova, Z; Adamkova, V; Poledne, R. Sex-specific interaction between APOE and APOA5 variants and determination of plasma lipid levels. *European Journal of Human Genetics,* 2008, 16, 135-138.

[65]Imbeault, P; Almeras, N; Richard, D; Despres, JP; Tremblay, A; Mauriege, P. Effect of a moderate weight loss on adipose tissue lipoprotein lipase activity and expression: existence of sexual variation and regional differences. *Int J Obes Relat Metab Disord,* 1999, 23(9), 957-65.

[66]Innis, SM; Hamilton, JJ. Effects, of developmental changes and early nutrition on cholesterol metabolism in infancy: a review. *J Am Coll Nutr.,* 1992, 11 Suppl, 63S-68S.

[67]Isaacs, A; Sayed-Tabatabaei, FA; Njajou, OT; Witteman, JC; Van Duijn, CM. The -514 C-T hepatic lipase promoter region polymorphism and plasma lipids: a meta-analysis. *J Clin Endocrinol Metab,* 2004, 89(8), 3858-63.

[68]Jansson, T; Powell, TL. Role of the placenta in fetal programming: underlying mechanisms and potential interventional approaches. *Clin Sci (Lond).,* 2007, 113(1), 1-13.

[69]Jensen, MD. Gender differences in regional fatty acid metabolism before and after meal ingestion. *Journal of Clinical Investigation.,* 1995, 96, 2297-2303.

[70]Karpe, F; Olivecrona, T; Olivecrona, G; Samra, JS; Summers, LK; Humphreys, SM., et al. Lipoprotein lipase transport in plasma: role of muscle and adipose tissues in regulation of plasma lipoprotein lipase concentrations. *J Lipid Res.,* 1998, 39(12), 2387-93.

[71]Kelishadi, R; Badiee, Z; Adeli, K. Cord bood lipid profile and associated factors: baseline data of a birth cohort study. *Paediatric and Perinatal Epidemiology,* 2007, 21, 518-524.

[72]Khan, QH; Pontefract, DE; Iyengar, S; Ye, S. Evidence of differing genotypic effects of PPARalpha in women and men. *J Med Genet.,* 2004, 41(6), e79.

[73]Khaw, KT; Barrett-Connor, E. Endogenous sex hormones, high density lipoprotein cholesterol, and other lipoprotein fractions in men. *Arterioscler Thromb,* 1991, 11(3), 489-94.

[74]Klaus, S; Keijer, J. Gene expression profiling of adipose tissue: individual, depot-dependent, and sex-dependent variabilities. *Nutrition*, 2004, 20(1), 115-20.

[75]Kleemola, P; Freese, R; Jauhiainen, M; Pahlman, R; Alfthan, G; Mutanen, M. Dietary determinants of serum paraoxonase activity in healthy humans. *Atherosclerosis*, 2002, 160(2), 425-32.

[76]Knuth, ND; Horowitz, JF. The elevation of ingested lipids within plasma chylomicrons is prolonged in men compared with women. *J Nutr.*, 2006, 136(6), 1498-503.

[77]Kotani, K; Sakane, N; Saiga, K; Adachi, S; Shimohiro, H; Mu, H., et al. Relationship between A-3826G polymorphism in the promoter of the uncoupling protein-1 gene and high-density lipoprotein cholesterol in Japanese individuals: a cross-sectional study. *Arch Med Res.,* 2008, 39(1), 142-6.

[78]Kotani, K; Sakane, N; Saiga, K; Tsuzaki, K; Shimohiro, H; Tabata, M., et al. The uncoupling protein-1 gene -3826A/G polymorphism and hypertension in Japanese subjects. *Clin Chem Lab Med.,* 2007, 45(9), 1186-9.

[79]Krauss, RM. Atherogenic lipoprotein phenotype and diet-gene interactions. *J Nutr.*, 2001, 131(2), 340S-3S.

[80]Kuk, JL; Lee, S; Heymsfield, SB; Ross, R. Waist circumference and abdominal adipose tissue distribution: influence of age and sex. *Am J Clin Nutr.,* 2005, 81(6), 1330-4.

[81]Kuzawa, CW; Adair, LS. Lipid profiles in adolescent Filipinos: relation to birth weight and maternal energy status during pregnancy. *Am J Clin Nutr.,* 2003, 77(4), 960-6.

[82]Kuzawa, CW; Adair, LS. A supply-demand model of fetal energy sufficiency predicts lipid profiles in male but not female Filipino adolescents. *Eur J Clin Nutr.,* 2004, 58(3), 438-48.

[83]Lamont, LS; McCullough, AJ; Kalhan, SC. Gender differences in the regulation of amino acid metabolism. *J Appl Physiol.,* 2003, 95(3), 1259-65.

[84]Lappas, M; Yee, K; Permezel, M; Rice, GE. Release and regulation of leptin, resistin and adiponectin from human placenta, fetal membranes, and maternal adipose tissue and skeletal muscle from normal and gestational diabetes mellitus-complicated pregnancies. *J Endocrinol.,* 2005, 186(3), 457-65.

[85]Lawlor, D; Ebrahim, S; Smith, GD. Sex matters: secular and geographical trends in sex differences in coronary heart disease and mortality. *BMJ*, 2001, 323, 541-545.

[86]Lawlor, D; Owen, CG; Davies, AA; Whincup, PH; Ebrahim, S; Cook, DG., et al. Sex differences in the association between birth weight and total cholesterol. *Annals of Epidemiology,* 2006, 16, 19-25.

[87]Le NaW, MF. Intrinsic enzymes of high-density lipoprotein. *Journal of Clinical Lipidology,* 2007, 1, 20-30.

[88]Legato, M. Gender-specific aspects of human biology. Amonk: *Futura Publishing Co. Inc.,* 1997.

[89]Leppaluoto, J; Hassi, J. Physiological adaptation of humans to the Finnish climate. In: J H, editor. Cold Climate Research in Finland. Helsinki: *Finnish Government Printing Centre.,* 1989. p. 18-26.

[90]Lewis, GF; Rader, DJ. New insights into the regulation of HDL metabolism and reverse cholesterol transport. *Circ Res.,* 2005, 96(12), 1221-32.

[91]Lindsay, RS; Walker, JD; Havel, PJ; Hamilton, BA; Calder, AA; Johnstone, FD. Adiponectin is present in cord blood but is unrelated to birth weight. *Diabetes Care,* 2003, 26(8), 2244-9.

[92]Lovegrove, JA; Gitau, R. Nutrigenetics and CVD: what does the future hold? *Proc Nutr Soc.,* 2008, 67(2), 206-13.

[93]Luczak ED and Leinward, LA. Sex-based cardiac physiology. *Annu Rev Physiol,* 2009, 71, 1-18.

[94]Luukkaa, V; Pesonen, U; Huhtaniemi, I; Lehtonen, A; Tilvis, R; Tuomilehto, J; et al. Inverse correlation between serum testosterone and leptin in men. *J Clin Endocrinol Metab.,* 1998, 83(9), 3243-6.

[95]Mahley, RW, Innerarity, TL; Rall, SC., Jr., Weisgraber KH. Plasma lipoproteins: apolipoprotein structure and function. *J Lipid Res.,* 1984, 25(12), 1277-94.

[96]Margetic, S; Gazzola, C; Pegg, GG; Hill, RA. Leptin: a review of its peripheral actions and interactions. *Int J Obes Relat Metab Disord,* 2002, 26(11), 1407-33.

[97]Martini, C., and Pallotini, VP. Cholesterol: from feeding to gene regulatin. *Genes Nutr.,* 2007, 2(2), 181-193.

[98]Masson, LF; McNeill, G; Avenell, A. Genetic variation and the lipid response to dietary intervention: a systematic review. *Am J Clin Nutr.,* 2003, 77(5), 1098-111.

[99]Matsubara, M; Maruoka, S; Katayose, S. Inverse relationship between plasma adiponectin and leptin concentrations in normal-weight and obese women. *Eur J Endocrinol,* 2002, 147(2), 173-80.

[100] McKeigue, PM; Laws, A; Chen, YD; Marmot, MG; Reaven, GM. Relation of plasma triglyceride and apoB levels to insulin-mediated suppression of nonesterified fatty acids. Possible explanation for sex differences in lipoprotein pattern. *Arterioscler Thromb,* 1993, 13(8), 1187-92.

[101] Meier, U; Gressner, AM. Endocrine regulation of energy metabolism: review of pathobiochemical and clinical chemical aspects of leptin, ghrelin, adiponectin, and resistin. *Clin Chem.,* 2004, 50(9), 1511-25.

[102] Memisoglu, A ; Hu, FB ; Hankinson, SE ; Manson, JE ; De Vivo, I ; Willett, WC., et al. Interaction between a peroxisome proliferator-activated receptor gamma gene polymorphism and dietary fat intake in relation to body mass. *Hum Mol Genet.,* 2003, 12(22), 2923-9.

[103] Mitchell, M, Armstrong, DT; Robker, RL; Norman, RJ. Adipokines: implications for female fertility and obesity. *Reproduction,* 2005, 130(5), 583-97.

[104] Mittendorfer, B. Sexual dimorphism in human lipid metabolism. *J Nutr.,* 2005, 135(4), 681-6.

[105] Mosher, MJ; Comuzzie; AG; Jett, K; Melvin, K; Rubica, R; Zlojutro, M; Crawford, MH. Evidence of sex-specific influence of adiponecting on HDL variation: The Kansas Nutrition Project. In: AAPA. Milwaukee: *Am. J. Physiocl Anthropology Suppl.,* 40:151, 2005.

[106] Mosher, MJ; Sorensen, MV; Leonard, WH. Nutrition and lipids in a population exhibiting very low levels of serum cholesterol: The Western Buryat of Ust Orda, Siberia. In: AAPA: 4th Wiley-Liss Symposium: Human populations of circumpolar regions: origins, adaptation and disease; 2006, *AJPA*, 2006.

[107] Mosher, MJ; Demarchi, DA; Crawford, MH. Genetic and environmental factors underlying sexual dimorphism in serum lipids: The Kansas Nutrition Project. In: Xth Latin American Congress on *Biological Anthropology;* 2008; La Plata, Argentina, 2008.

[108] Mosher, MJ; Lange, LA; Howard, BV; Lee, ET; Best, LG; Fabsitz, RR., et al. Sex-specific interaction between APOE genotype and carbohydrate intake affects plasma HDL-C levels: the Strong Heart Family Study. *Genes Nutr.,* 2008, 3(2), 87-97.

[109] Mosher, MJ; Martin, LJ; Cupples, LA; Yang, Q; Dyer, TD; Williams, JT., et al. Genotype-by-sex interaction in the regulation of high-density lipoprotein: the Framingham Heart Study. *Hum Biol.,* 2005, 77(6), 773-93.

[110] Myant, N. Cholesterol Metabolism, LDL and teh LDL Receptor. San Diego: Academic Press, Inc; 1990.

[111] Myatt, L. Placental adaptive responses and fetal programming. *J Physiol,* 2006, 572 (Pt 1), 25-30.

[112] Nakamura, MT; Cheon, Y; Li, Y; Nara, TY. Mechanisms of regulation of gene expression by fatty acids. *Lipids*, 2004, 39(11), 1077-83.

[113] Nelson, SM; Freeman, DJ; Sattar, N; Johnstone, FD; Lindsay, RS. IGF-1 and leptin associate with fetal HDL cholesterol at birth: examination in offspring of mothers with type 1 diabetes. *Diabetes*, 2007, 56(11), 2705-9.

[114] Nijland, MJ; Ford, SP; Nathanielsz, PW. Prenatal origins of adult disease. *Curr Opin Obstet Gynecol,* 2008, 20(2), 132-8.

[115] Nindl, BC; Scoville, CR; Sheehan, KM; Leone, CD; Mello, RP. Gender differences in regional body composition and somatotrophic influences of IGF-I and leptin. *J Appl Physiol,* 2002, 92(4), 1611-8.

[116] Norgan, NG. The beneficial effects of body fat and adipose tissue in humans. *Int J Obes Relat Metab Disord,* 1997, 21(9), 738-46.

[117] North, KE; Franceschini, N; Borecki, IB; Gu, CC; Heiss, G; Province, MA., et al. Genotype-by-sex interaction on fasting insulin concentration: the HyperGEN study. *Diabetes,* 2007, 56(1), 137-42.

[118] Oh, HH; Kim, KS; Choi, SM; Yang, HS; Yoon, Y. The effects of uncoupling protein-1 genotype on lipoprotein cholesterol level in Korean obese subjects. *Metabolism*, 2004, 53(8), 1054-9.

[119] Ong, K; Frystyk, J; Flyvbjerg, A; Petry, CJ. Avon Longitudinal Study of Parents and Childrens Study Team, A Ness and DB Dunger. Sex-discordant associations with adiponecting levels and lipid profiles in children. *Diabetes*, 2006, 55, 1137-1341.

[120] Ordovas, JM and Corrella, C. Genes, diet and plasma lipids: the evidence from observational studies. In: Simopoulos AaJO, editor. *Nutrigenetics and Nutrigenomics.* Basel: Karger, 2004.

[121] Ordovas, JM. Gender, a significant factor in the cross talk between genes, environment, and health. *Gend Med.,* 2007, 4 Suppl B:S111-22.

[122] Ordovas, JM; Corella, D; Demissie, S; Cupples, LA; Couture, P; Coltell, O., et al. Dietary fat intake determines the effect of a common polymorphism in the hepatic lipase gene promoter on high-density lipoprotein metabolism: evidence of a strong dose effect in this gene-nutrient interaction in the Framingham Study. *Circulation*, 2002, 106(18), 2315-21.

[123] Owen, CG; Whincup, PH; Odoki, K; Gilg, JA; Cook, DG. Birth weight and blood cholesterol level: a study in adolescents and systematic review. *Pediatrics*, 2003, 111(5 Pt 1), 1081-9.

[124] Pac-Kozuchowska. Evaluation of lipids, lipoproteins and apolipoproteins concentration in cord blood serum of newborns from rural and urban environments. *Ann Aggric Environ Med.,* 2007, 14, 25-29.

[125] Paracchini, V; Pedotti, P; Taioli, E. Genetics of leptin and obesity: a HuGE review. *Am J Epidemiol.,* 2005, 162(2), 101-14.

[126] Patsopoulos, NA; Tatsioni, A; Ioannidis, JP. Claims of sex differences: an empirical assessment in genetic associations. *Jama*, 2007, 298(8), 880-93.

[127] Pepe, GJ. and Albrecht, ED. Actions of placental and fetal adrenal steroid hormones in primate pregnancy. *Endocrine review*, 1995, 16(5), 608-648.

[128] Phillips, S. Protein metabolism and exercise: potential sex-based differences. In: Tarnopolsky M; editor. Gender differences in metabolism: practical and nutritional implications. *Boca Raton:* CRC Press; 1999. p. 155-178.

[129] Pietrobelli, A; Allison, DB; Heshka, S; Heo, M; Wang, ZM; Bertkau, A., et al. Sexual dimorphism in the energy content of weight change. *Int J Obes Relat Metab Disord,* 2002, 26(10), 1339-48.

[130] Pilote, L; Dasgupta, K; Guru, V; Humphries, KH; McGrath, J; Norris, C., et al. A comprehensive view of sex-specific issues related to cardiovascular disease. *Cmaj*, 2007, 176(6), S1-44.

[131] Power, ML; Schulkin, J. Sex differences in fat storage, fat metabolism, and the health risks from obesity: possible evolutionary origins. *Br J Nutr*., 2008, 99(5), 931-40.

[132] Qi, L; Shen, H; Larson, I; Barnard, JR; Schaefer, EJ; Ordovas, JM. Genetic variation at the hormone sensitive lipase: gender-specific association with plasma lipid and glucose concentrations. *Clin Genet,* 2004, 65(2), 93-100.

[133] Rainey, WE; Parker, CR; Jr., Rehman, K; Carr, BR. The adrenal genetic puzzle: how do the fetal and adult pieces differ? *Endocr Res.,* 2002, 28(4), 611-22.

[134] Rantala, M; Silaste, ML; Tuominen, A; Kaikkonen, J; Salonen, JT; Alfthan, G., et al. Dietary modifications and gene polymorphisms alter serum paraoxonase activity in healthy women. *J Nutr*., 2002, 132(10), 3012-7.

[135] Rees, WD; McNeil, CJ; Maloney, CA. The Roles of PPARs in the Fetal Origins of Metabolic Health and Disease. *PPAR Res*., 2008, 2008, 459030.

[136] Reik, W; Constancia, M; Fowden, A; Anderson, N; Dean, W; Ferguson-Smith, A., et al. Regulation of supply and demand for maternal nutrients in mammals by imprinted genes. *J Physiol*., 2003, 547(Pt 1), 35-44.

[137] Rodriguez, AM; Palou, A. Uncoupling proteins: gender dependence and their relation to body weight control. *Int J Obes Relat Metab Disord.,* 2004, 28(4), 500-2.

[138] Ronti, T; Lupattelli, G; Mannarino, E. The endocrine function of adipose tissue: an update. *Clin Endocrinol (Oxf),* 2006, 64(4), 355-65.

[139] Rozek, LS; Hatsukami, TS; Richter, RJ; Ranchalis, J; Nakayama, K; McKinstry, LA., et al. The correlation of paraoxonase (PON1) activity with lipid and lipoprotein levels differs with vascular disease status. *J Lipid Res*., 2005, 46(9), 1888-95.

[140] Ruby B. Gender differences in carbohydrate metabolism: rest, exercise, and post exercise. In: Tarnopolsky M, editor. Gender difference in metabolism: practical and nutritional implications. *Boca Raton*: CRC Press, 1999, p. 121-154.

[141] Sagoo, GS; Tatt, I; Salanti, G; Butterworth, AS; Sarwar, N; Van Maarle, M., et al. Seven lipoprotein lipase gene polymorphisms, lipid fractions, and coronary disease: a HuGE association review and meta-analysis. *Am J Epidemiol*, 2008, 168(11), 1233-46.

[142] Scanu, AM; Edelstein, C. HDL: bridging past and present with a look at the future. *Faseb J*., 2008, 22(12), 4044-54.

[143] Schooling, CM; Lam, TH; Thomas, GN; Cowling, BJ; Heys, M; Janus, ED., et al. Growth environment and sex differences in lipids, body shape and diabetes risk. PLoS ONE, 2007, 2(10), e1070.

[144] Schubring, C; Kiess, W; Englaro, P; Rascher, W; Dotsch, J; Hanitsch, S., et al. Levels of leptin in maternal serum, amniotic fluid, and arterial and venous cord blood: relation to neonatal and placental weight. *J Clin Endocrinol Metab.,* 1997, 82(5), 1480-3.

[145] Senti, M; Tomas, M; Elosual, R; Sala, J; Masia, R; Marrugat, J. The paraoxonase-1 codon 192 polymorphism is associated with fasting total cholesterol and LDL-cholesterol concentrations only in postmenopausal women. The REGICOR study. *Clin Chem Lab Med.,* 2002, 40(7), 677-83.

[146] Shi, J; Simpkins, JW. 17 beta-Estradiol modulation of glucose transporter 1 expression in blood-brain barrier. *Am J Physiol,* 1997, 272(6 Pt 1), E1016-22.

[147] Simoneau, JA; Bouchard, C. Genetic determinism of fiber type proportion in human skeletal muscle. *Faseb J.,* 1995, 9(11), 1091-5.

[148] Skidmore, PM; Cassidy, A; Swaminathan, R; Falchi, M; Spector, TD, MacGregor, AJ. Intrauterine, environmental, and genetic influences in the relationship between birth weight and lipids in a female twin cohort. *Arterioscler Thromb Vasc Biol.,* 2006, 26(10), 2373-9.

[149] Skidmore, PM, Hardy, RJ; Kuh, DJ; Langenberg, C, Wadsworth, ME. Birth weight and lipids in a national birth cohort study. *Arterioscler Thromb Vasc Biol.,* 2004, 24(3), 588-94.

[150] Sneider, H. The age dependency of gene expression for plasma lipids, lipoproteins and apolipoproteins. *Am J Hum Genet,* 1997, 60, 638-650.

[151] Snieder, H; Van Doornen, LJ; Boomsma, DI. Dissecting the genetic architecture of lipids, lipoproteins, and apolipoproteins: lessons from twin studies. *Arterioscler Thromb Vasc Biol.,* 1999, 19(12), 2826-34.

[152] Stengard, JH; Clark, AG; Weiss, KM; Kardia, S; Nickerson, DA; Salomaa, V., et al. Contributions of 18 additional DNA sequence variations in the gene encoding apolipoprotein E to explaining variation in quantitative measures of lipid metabolism. *Am J Hum Genet.,* 2002, 71(3), 501-17.

[153] Talmud, PJ; Palmen, J; Luan, J; Flavell, D; Byrne, CD; Waterworth, DM., et al. Variation in the promoter of the human hormone sensitive lipase gene shows gender specific effects on insulin and lipid levels: results from the Ely study. *Biochim Biophys Acta,* 2001, 1537(3), 239-44.

[154] Tarnopolsky, M. Females and males; should nutritional recommendations be gender specific? *Sportmedizin und Sporttraumatologie,* 2003, 51(1), 39-46.

[155] Tarnopolsky, MaRC. Hormonal differences between males and females. In: Tarnopolsky M, editor. Gender differences in metabolism: practical and nutritional implications. Baton Rouge: CRC Press; 1999. p. 1-35.

[156] Thomas-Moya, E; Gianotti, M; Proenza, AM; Llado, I. Paraoxonase 1 response to a high-fat diet: gender differences in the factors involved. *Mol Med.,* 2007, 13(3-4), 203-9.

[157] Tome, MA; Lage, M; Camina, JP; Garcia-Mayor, RV; Dieguez, C, Casanueva, FF. Sex-based differences in serum leptin concentrations from umbilical cord blood at delivery. *Eur J Endocrinol,* 1997, 137(6), 655-8.

[158] Tsuchida, A; Yamauchi, T; Takekawa, S; Hada, Y; Ito, Y; Maki, T., et al. Peroxisome proliferator-activated receptor (PPAR)alpha activation increases adiponectin receptors and reduces obesity-related inflammation in adipose tissue: comparison of activation of PPARalpha, PPARgamma, and their combination. *Diabetes*, 2005, 54(12), 3358-70.

[159] Uhi-Bronner, S; Waltisperger, E; Martinez-Lorenzana, G; Condes Lara, M; Freund-Mercier MJ. Sexually dimorphic expression of oxytocin binding sites in forebrain and spinal cord of the rat. *Neuroscience*, 2005, 135(1), 147-54.
[160] Valle A; Santandreu, FM; Garcia-Palmer, FJ; Roca, P; Oliver, J. The serum levels of 17beta-estradiol, progesterone and triiodothyronine correlate with brown adipose tissue thermogenic parameters during aging. *Cell Physiol Biochem,* 2008, 22(1-4), 337-46.
[161] Voet, D; Voet, J. Lipids and membranes. In: Biochemistry. First Edition ed. New York: Wiley and Sons, 1990.
[162] Votruba, SB; Jensen, MD. Regional fat deposition as a factor in FFA metabolism. *Annu Rev Nutr.,* 2007, 27, 149-63.
[163] Votruba, SB; Jensen, MD. Sex differences in abdominal, gluteal, and thigh LPL activity. *Am J Physiol Endocrinol Metab.,* 2007, 292(6), E1823-8.
[164] Wang, J; Thornton, JC; Russell, M; Burastero, S; Heymsfield, S; Pierson, RN., Jr. Asians have lower body mass index (BMI) but higher percent body fat than do whites: comparisons of anthropometric measurements. *Am J Clin Nutr.,* 1994, 60(1), 23-8.
[165] Weggemans, RM; Zock, PL; Ordovas, JM; Ramos-Galluzzi, J; Katan, MB. Genetic polymorphisms and lipid response to dietary changes in humans. *Eur J Clin Invest,* 2001, 31(11), 950-7.
[166] Weinberg, SL. The diet-heart hypothesis: a critique. *J Am Coll Cardiol,* 2004, 43(5), 731-3.
[167] Weiss, K. Genetic variation and human disease: Principles and evolutionary approaches. Cambridge: Cambridge University Press, 1993.
[168] Weiss, LA; Pan, L; Abney, M; Ober, C. The sex-specific genetic architecture of quantitative traits in humans. *Nat Genet,* 2006, 38(2), 218-22.
[169] Welle, S; Tawil, R; Thornton, CA. Sex-related differences in gene expression in human skeletal muscle. PLoS ONE, 2008, 3(1), e1385.
[170] Wells, JC. Sexual dimorphism of body composition. *Best Pract Res Clin Endocrinol Metab.,* 2007, 21(3), 415-30.
[171] Wenk, MR. The emerging field of lipidomics. *Nat Rev Drug Discov,* 2005, 4(7), 594-610.
[172] Werko, L. End of the road for the diet-heart theory? *Scand Cardiovasc J,* 2008, 42(4), 250-5.
[173] Wiecek, A; Adamczak, M; Chudek, J. Adiponectin--an adipokine with unique metabolic properties. *Nephrol Dial Transplant,* 2007, 22(4), 981-8.
[174] Williams, CM. Lipid metabolism in women. *Proc Nutr Soc.,* 2004, 63(1), 153-60.
[175] Winnier, D; Rainwater, DL; Cole, SA; Williams, JT; Dyer, TD; Blangero, J; MacCluer, JW; Mahaney, MC. Sex-specific QTL effects on variation in paraoxonase 1 (PON1) activity in Mexican Americans. *Genetic Epidemiology,* 200, 31, 66-74.
[176] Wizemannn, TM and Pardue, MP., eds. Exploring the biological contributions human health: does sex matter? Washington: *National Academy Press,* 2001.
[177] Woods, SC; Gotoh, K; Clegg, DJ. Gender differences in the control of energy homeostasis. *Exp Biol Med (Maywood),* 2003; 228(10); 1175-80.
[178] Woollett, LA. Fetal lipid metabolism. *Front Biosci,* 2001; 6; D536-45.
[179] Woollett, LA. Maternal cholesterol in fetal development: transport of cholesterol from the maternal to the fetal circulation. *Am J Clin Nutr.,* 2005, 82(6), 1155-61.

[180] Woollett, LA. Where does fetal and embryonic cholesterol originate and what does it do? *Annu Rev Nutr.,* 2008, 28, 97-114.
[181] Yamauchi, T; Kamon, J; Minokoshi, Y; Ito, Y; Waki, H; Uchida, S., et al. Adiponectin stimulates glucose utilization and fatty-acid oxidation by activating AMP-activated protein kinase. *Nat Med.,* 2002, 8(11), 1288-95.
[182] Ye, SQ; Kwiterovich, PO., Jr. Influence of genetic polymorphisms on responsiveness to dietary fat and cholesterol. *Am J Clin Nutr.,* 2000, 72(5 Suppl), 1275S-1284S.
[183] Yeagle, PL. Roles of cholesterol in cellular functions. In: Eshahani MaJS, editor. *Advances in cholesterol research. Philadelphia:* Telford Press, 1990.
[184] Yost, TJ; Jensen, DR; Haugen, BR; Eckel, RH. Effect of dietary macronutrient composition on tissue-specific lipoprotein lipase activity and insulin action in normal-weight subjects. *Am J Clin Nutr.,* 1998, 68(2), 296-302.
[185] Yu, YH; Ginsberg, HN. Adipocyte signaling and lipid homeostasis: sequelae of insulin-resistant adipose tissue. *Circ Res.,* 2005, 96(10), 1042-52.

In: Nutritional Education
Editor: Ida R. Laidyth

ISBN: 978-1-60876-078-7

Chapter 5

METABOLIC SYNDROME IN CHILDREN: PROMOTING HEALTH, FITNESS AND WELLNESS IN ELEMENTARY SCHOOL CHILDREN

Millee Jorge[1] and Daniel H. Riddick[2]
[1]School of Physical Therapy Langston University, Langston Oklahoma, USA
[2]Department of Reproductive Endocrinology, University of Vermont, School of Medicine, Burlington, Vermont, USA

INTRODUCTION

The obesity epidemic in the United States and the continuing rise in the number of children and adolescents who are overweight and have type 2 diabetes mellitus[1], as well as reports by life-course epidemiologists [2] who identify that poor health in childhood can lead to acute and chronic illness in adulthood, provide evidence that the presence of metabolic syndrome in children and adolescents is a risk factor for developing cardiovascular disease and type 2 diabetes[3]. The purpose of this paper is threefold: (1) To review the risk factors for developing metabolic syndrome in children and adolescents; (2) to report on the projected long-term health effects of metabolic syndrome; and (3) to describe health and wellness programs that have been implemented to address the rise in overweight children and adolescents at risk for metabolic syndrome, cardiovascular disease, and type 2 diabetes mellitus.

DEFINING METABOLIC SYNDROME

Metabolic Syndrome X was first described by Dr. Gerald Reaven in 1988 when he published, "Role of insulin resistance in human disease"[4]. Reaven described how the presence of insulin resistance and the body's compensatory response of hyperinsulinemia may avoid the development of hyperglycemia but can create a host of pathologic conditions including: (1) glucose intolerance, (2) high levels of plasma triglycerides, (3) low density lipoprotein cholesterol, and (4) hypertension. The presentation of these health conditions as a cluster of abnormal findings in the presence of insulin resistance was termed Metabolic Syndrome X. [4] The significance of Metabolic Syndrome X was initially related to cardiovascular disease risk and later was expanded to include a risk factor for developing type 2 diabetes mellitus.

Since 1988 Reaven[5,6] , other researchers [7-9] as well as health entities such as The World Health Organization[10] and the National Cholesterol Education Program Adult Treatment Panel III (ATP III)[11] have investigated the relationship of metabolic syndrome to the development of co-morbidities.[12] Each has defined parameters for establishing whether an individual has metabolic syndrome. (Table 1) Although metabolic syndrome was initially reported in adults it is now alsocdescribed in children and adolescents. [2,3,9,13] There is currently, however, no consensus on the definition of metabolic syndrome in children[2]

For purposes of this paper, the definition of metabolic syndrome in children will be that of the Third Report of the National Cholesterol Education Program (Adult Treatment Panel III). [11] A child or adolescent with any three of the following conditions is said to have metabolic syndrome: (1) fasting glucose equal to or greater than 100mg/dL; (2) fasting triglycerides equal to or greater than 150mg/dL; (3) high density lipoprotein (HDL) cholesterol of less than 40 mg/dL or less in males and 50 mg/dL or less in females; (4) waist circumference greater than 102 cm in males or 88 cm in females; and (5) elevated systolic (≥130mmHg) and/or (≥85mmHg) diastolic blood pressure. Persons already being treated with medication for dyslipidemia, hypertension, and hyperglycemia are included in the cluster of diagnostic categories.

Table 1. Comparison of Metabolic Syndrome Definition

Cluster of symptoms	World Health Organization	National Cholesterol Education Panel (Adult Treatment Panel III)
	One of the following:	Any three of the following
Type 2 Diabetes Mellitus	Type 2 diabetes mellitus	Treatment for type 2 diabetes mellitus
Impaired fasting glucose	Impaired fasting glucose 110-125 mg/dL	Impaired fasting glucose ≥110 mg/dL
Impaired fasting glucose tolerance test	Impaired fasting glucose tolerance test 140-199mg/dL	Treatment for elevated glucose
Insulin resistance	Insulin resistance	
	Any two of the following:	
Hypertension	Hypertension 130/85 mmHg	Hypertension 130/85 mmHg
Elevated triglycerides	Elevated triglycerides—150 mg/dL or greater	Fasting triglycerides ≥150 mg/dL
High density lipoprotein (HDL) Cholesterol	HDL lower than 35 mg/dL in men and 39 mg/dL in women	HDL <40mg/dL in men and<50mg/dL in women
Body Mass Index (BMI)	Body mass index (BMI) greater than 30kg/m^2	
Abdominal or central adiposity	Waist to hip ratio .9 or greater in men and .85 or greater in women	Waist circumference greater than 102 cm in men and 88 cm in women

EPIDEMIOLOGY

The United States is experiencing an epidemic of obesity in the adult population with greater than 66% of adults reported to be overweight or obese[14] as reported by the Centers for Disease Control and Prevention (CDC) National Center for Health Statistics (NCHS) and based on the results of the 2003-2004 comparison data from the National Health and Nutrition Examination Survey (NHANES). Researchers [13,14,16] report that the number of children and adolescents who are overweight or obese has tripled in the last three decades. The CDC NCHS report that 17% of children and adolescents 2-19 years of age in the United States are overweight. Overweight in children is defined as a body mass index (BMI) ≥85th percentile but < 95th percentile. Obesity is defined as a BMI ≥ 95th percentile. [12]

In a study by Duncan, Sierra, and Xiao-Hua [13] researchers used the NHANES data to look for overall prevalence of metabolic syndrome in children and adolescents. They reported 4.2% of 12-19 year olds had metabolic syndrome based on NHANES III data collected during 1988-1994. The number of children and adolescents with metabolic syndrome increased to 6.4% in NHANES IV data collected during 1999-2000. Thirty-two percent of overweight adolescents had metabolic syndrome. The researchers reported an estimate of 2 million U.S. adolescents who have metabolic syndrome.

HEALTH CONDITIONS FOR WHICH METABOLIC SYNDROME IS A RISK FACTOR

Based on the abnormal changes noted in the health factors (blood pressure, cholesterol, glucose levels, central adiposity, BMI) that are included in the definition for metabolic syndrome by the World Health Organization[10] or the National Cholesterol Education Program Adult Treatment Panel III,[11] persons with the metabolic syndrome are at risk for other health related conditions: obesity[18], cardiovascular disease[19], type 2 diabetes mellitus[12], non-alcoholic fatty liver disease[20], and polycystic ovarian syndrome[1]. Evaluating children and adolescents for metabolic syndrome could identify those individuals at risk for chronic health conditions and decrease the occurrence of these conditions in later years.

OBESITY IN CHILDHOOD AND ADOLESCENCE

Monitoring weight, BMI and waist circumference in children and adolescents is a health-targeted strategy that can identify children at risk for metabolic syndrome. Hirschler et al. (2007)[15] reported anthropometric measurements of 5103 children 4-13 years of age. The results of the study revealed that 6.0% of the students were obese with a BMI ≥95th percentile; 13.6% were overweight with a BMI ≥85th percentile up to the 94th percentile; and 80.4 % were non-overweight with a BMI < 85th percentile. The researchers concluded that waist circumference and BMI predict metabolic syndrome in children[15]. Waist circumference equal to or greater than the 75th percentile may be the threshold that best describes the child with metabolic syndrome.

Hirschler et al. [15] also evaluated blood glucose levels, lipid profiles, and insulin assay results in 530 children in the study. They reported metabolic syndrome was present in 31% of children and adolescents with BMI in the 95th percentile or higher, 22% of children and adolescents with BMI in overweight range—85th-94th percentile range, and 6% in non-overweight children and adolescents.

The Princeton Lipid Research Clinic [21] follow-up study that included children and adolescents ages 6-19, published in the journal of *Pediatrics* in 2007, reported that an increase in age-specific BMI percentile from childhood to adulthood was a significant predictor of cardiovascular disease. The researchers recommended that evaluating children and adolescents for metabolic syndrome could identify those individuals at risk for adult cardiovascular disease.

ELEVATED BLOOD PRESSURE

The Fourth Report on the Diagnosis, Evaluation, and Treatment of High Blood Pressure in Children and Adolescents: The National High Blood Pressure Education Program Working Group on High Blood Pressure in Children and Adolescents [19] revised the blood pressure tables to include 50th, 90th, 95th and 99th percentiles by gender, age and height.

http://www.nhlbi.nih.gov/guidelines/hypertension/child_tbl.pdf (Appendix 1). Hypertension is defined as systolic pressure and/or diastolic blood pressure that on repeated measure is ≥95th percentile. Children with blood pressure in the 90th-94th percentile have pre-hypertension and children and with blood pressure at the 95th percentile or higher have hypertension[19].

In a study by Paradis G. et al.[22] "Blood Pressure and Adiposity in Children and Adolescents" published in the Journal *Circulation* in 2004, the researchers reported 12% of 9-year-old males, 22% of 13-year-old males, and 30% of 16-year-old males had hypertension. Females in the study were also found to have hypertension: 14% of 9-year-old females, 19% of 13-year-old females, and 17% of 16-year-old females.

CARDIOVASCULAR DISEASE

The National Institutes of Health—National Heart, Lung, and Blood Institute Lipid Research conducted a prevalence study in 1973-1976 and a follow-up study in 2000-2004. Researchers reported "Metabolic syndrome in childhood predicts adult cardiovascular disease 25 years later" [21]. Metabolic syndrome in children and adolescents proved to be a significant predictor for cardiovascular disease in adulthood.

The SEARCH for Diabetes in Youth Study[23] has issued reports that children and adolescents with diabetes mellitus are at risk for cardiovascular disease. Cardiovascular disease factors are implicated in each of the major disease co-morbidities that arise from the cluster of symptoms that is defined as metabolic syndrome.

Diabetes Mellitus in Children and Adolescents

In the past two decades the incidence of diabetes in children and adolescents has been estimated to have increased 20-fold.[19] This alarming estimate includes a dramatic increase in children with type 1 diabetes mellitus, and an increase in the number of children and adolescents with type 2 diabetes. The rise of type 2 diabetes, a disease that was previously typically described as a disease of adult onset, and the increase incidence of type I diabetes mellitus, prompted the Centers for Disease Control and Prevention and the National Institute of Diabetes and Digestive and Kidney Diseases to fund a multi-center study: "SEARCH for Diabetes in Youth"[23] that began with a 5-year grant cycle (phase 1) in 2002 and is continuing with another 5 year cycle that began in 2006-2010 (phase 2). As reported on the SEARCH website, http://www.searchfordiabetes.org/public/provider/index.cfm ,

The study goals are to:

"(1) Identify the number of children and youth under age 20 who have diabetes, (2) study how type 1 diabetes and type 2 diabetes differ, including how they differ by age and race/ethnicity, (3) learn more about the complications of diabetes in children and youth, (4) investigate the different types of care and medical treatment that these children and youth receive, and (5) learn more about how diabetes affects the everyday lives of children and youth who have diabetes." [23]

In 2001, the incidence of physician-diagnosed diabetes mellitus in children and adolescents was reported as one in every 523 persons 20 years and younger in the United States.[23] 154,000 of the 81 million children and adolescents in the United States had diabetes in 2001. [22] Rodriguez et al. [24] reported data from SEARCH for Diabetes in Youth Study, "Prevalence of cardiovascular disease risk factors in U.S. children and adolescents with diabetes" published in *Diabetes Care* (2006). 92% of children and adolescents with type 2 diabetes mellitus were found to have two other cardiovascular risk factors.

Metabolic syndrome is considered a risk factor for developing type 2 diabetes mellitus. Persons diagnosed with diabetes mellitus before 20 years of age have a lower life expectancy.[22] Therefore preventing metabolic syndrome in children is of paramount importance. Diagnosing and treating metabolic syndrome in children and adolescents can prevent the secondary risk factor of type 2 diabetes as well as associated cardiovascular disease risk factors.

Nonalcoholic Fatty Liver Disease

When children and adolescents have metabolic syndrome that is undiagnosed and untreated, chronic long-term changes occur in the liver. Metabolic syndrome is a risk factor for developing nonalcoholic fatty liver disease (NAFLD)[20]. Angulo[20] reports that obesity in childhood and adolescence contributes to NAFLD. Data indicates that one out of every 10 children/adolescents in the United States have NAFLD. Adams and Angulo[25] report that greater than ninety percent of persons with NAFLD have at least on feature of metabolic syndrome. Thirty percent of these individuals have nonalcoholic steatohepatitis (NASH)—a silent form of liver disease. NASH is fatty liver with an inflammatory process that causes tissue injury and scarring. Untreated NASH can lead to cirrhosis of the liver. Liver disease in children associated with obesity and metabolic syndrome has increased the need for liver transplantation in young adults.

POLYCYSTIC OVARIAN SYNDROME

The polycystic ovary syndrome (PCOS) was first described in 1935 by Stein and Leventhal.[26] They reported their findings in 7 women with oligomenorrhea, hirsutism, infertility and enlarged, anatomically polycystic ovaries. The condition was believed to be rare and a disorder of adult women. It is now recognized that PCOS is neither rare nor limited to adulthood. 6-8% of reproductive age women[27,28] and up to 10% of adolescents[29] exhibit the signs and symptoms of PCOS.

PCOS is the most common endocrine disorder in women, and its symptoms begin at or before puberty.[30-38] 55% of adolescents with irregular menses continuing more than 2 years after menarche have changes associated with PCOS.[39]

PCOS resembles closely the metabolic syndrome with additional findings related to increased androgen production. The incidence of metabolic syndrome in adolescent girls with PCOS has been reported to be 37% compared to 5% in control adolescents. [40]

As with metabolic syndrome, a number of definitions and diagnostic criteria have been proposed for PCOS. [41-43] The diagnostic criteria for PCOS most useful in the diagnosis and treatment of adolescents is that recommended by the Androgen Excess Society Task Force in 2006[43] and includes the elements seen in Table 2.

Table 2. Diagnostic Criteria for PCOS in Adolescents*

Hyperandrogenism	Clinical or Laboratory
Ovarian dysfunction	Irregular menses>2 years after menarche OR polycystic ovaries on ultrasonography
Exclusions of other androgen excess conditions including	Non-classical CAH (congenital adrenal hyperplasia, Cushing's syndrome, androgen producing neoplasm of ovary or adrenal

* Adapted from Androgen Excess Society Guidelines

The hormonal abnormalities underlying the clinical picture of PCOS are related in a cyclic fashion, such that it has not yet been possible to establish a single initial cause of the disorder. PCOS is a syndrome not a disease. It is apparent from a depiction of the hormonal interactions shown in Figure 1 that entry into this cycle of endocrinopathy can occur through several different portals.

There is a strong familial history of PCOS in some individuals but by no means in all. An underlying genetic abnormality affecting the function of enzymes involved in androgen production by both the ovaries and the adrenal glands has been reported. [44-47] Significant improvement in the condition has been reported following weight loss through diet and exercise in obese adults and adolescents with PCOS.[48-52] The prevalence of obesity in persons with PCOS has been reported to be between 40- 80%.[29,53,57-59[Thus, obesity may be the precipitating event in many persons who develop PCOS.

The severity of hirsutism, anovulation and insulin resistance in PCOS is directly related to the Body Mass Index (BMI).[53,29,54-56[It is now believed that insulin resistance is present in most adolescents with PCOS[40,60,61] and 33% have glucose intolerance.[62-64] Insulin resistance drives the increased androgen production responsible for hirsutism, anovulation, and difficulty with weight control seen in PCOS (Fig.1). The presence of acanthosis nigracans, velvety darkly pigmented areas in neck and axillary skin folds, is a marker of insulin resistance.

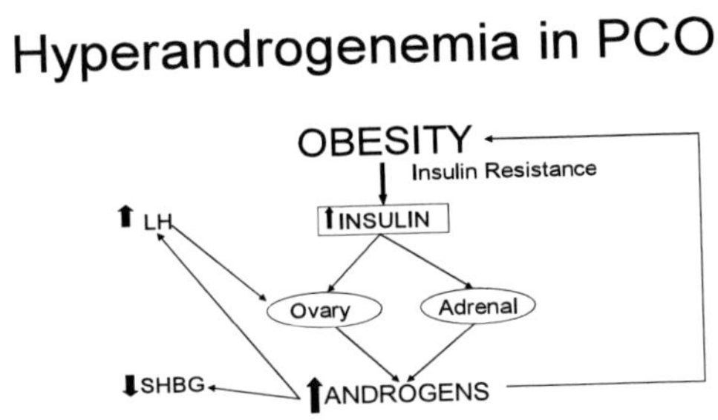

Figure 1. Interrelationships between obesity and hyperandrogenemia

There are major long term health risks of PCOS. Overall 40-74% of persons with PCOS have or will develop metabolic syndrome [40,62,65,66] as well as the later adult life sequellae of Type 2 diabetes [70-73], hypertension , dyslipidemia, cardiovascular disease and stroke. [67-69] The anovulation resulting in unopposed estrogen stimulation of the endometrium that accompanies both metabolic syndrome and PCOS puts such individuals at increased risk for the development of endometrial cancer at an early age.[74-76] Additionally, there are major psychosocial effects of obesity, compounded by the disfiguring presence of acne and excessive facial and body hair particularly upsetting to the adolescent.[77-79]

There is much overlap between adolescent obesity, PCOS, and metabolic syndrome. Whether these entities merely share certain signs and symptoms or are more closely connected through similar underlying pathophysiologic mechanisms and are thus variants of the same disorder awaits further study.

Treatment Guidelines for Children and Adolescents with Metabolic Syndrome

The medical community has not developed consensus on a specific definition for children and adolescents with metabolic syndrome, and there are currently no specific treatment guidelines for metabolic syndrome in children. However, the U.S. obesity epidemic, the rise in number of children and adolescents who are overweight or obese, the rise in the incidence of children and adolescents with diabetes mellitus, and other health concerns has prompted the development of treatment guidelines for prevention and treatment of obesity in the pediatric population. The guideline that will be presented was issued in 2008 by the Endocrine Society in the U.S.[17] and is based on expert opinion.

Prevention and Treatment of Pediatric Obesity Guideline

The Endocrine Society issued a Treatment Guideline for the prevention and treatment of pediatric obesity which was published in the Journal of Clinical Endocrinology and Metabolism in 2008. [17] The guidelines define overweight as those children and adolescents with a BMI $\geq 85^{th}$ percentile but $< 95^{th}$ percentile and obese as those children and adolescents having a BMI $\geq 95^{th}$ percentile.

For the prevention of overweight children the guideline proposes adhering to a healthy diet and engaging in daily physical exercise as fundamental to managing weight and prevention of primary and secondary problems such as metabolic syndrome. The guideline states that schools should provide a minimum of 60 minutes of moderate or vigorous exercise daily in all grades. The use of education as a means for promotion of good nutrition and physical exercise is essential within the school system and in communities at large.

In the treatment of children and adolescents who are overweight and obese and who may have other co-morbidities such as metabolic syndrome, the guideline advocates lifestyle modification as the first treatment approach. Life style modification in what children and adolescents eat: Alteration in diet from a high fat and high calorie diet to a low fat and low calorie diet; and life style modification in what children do for exercise: Increased activities to a daily exercise regimen that includes a minimum of 60 minutes of moderate to maximum intensity exercise is recommended.

The guideline recommends the use of pharmacological treatment in obese children only after lifestyle modification has failed to make a significant difference in the health of the child. In overweight children, pharmacological management should be considered only when there have been failed attempts at intensive life style modification and the child or adolescent has significant co-morbidities.

The guideline addresses the use of bariatric surgery in adolescents who have BMI over $50kg/m^2$ or $40kg/m^2$ and severe co-morbidities. Consideration of surgery should occur only after intensive lifestyle modification and pharmacological treatment have failed.

The guideline also addresses factors that have the potential to contribute to the prevention and treatment of pediatric obesity within the societal realm. There is the need to evaluate those factors that contribute to poor eating habits such as frequent and intensive exposure to unhealthy food choices through advertisement to children and to implement new regulations and policies that protect children. Non-nutritious and poor food and drink choices should be eliminated from the school environment. Communities need to come together to assure there are safe environments for physical activity for children. Health practitioners should advocate to policymakers regarding the need for all communities to have access to nutritious foods high in quality and freshness at affordable prices.

Interventions to Address the Growing Health Concerns of Children and Adolescents

The US Department of Health and Human Services in Healthy People 2010 [80] specifically addressed the desire to promote health and reduce chronic disease associated with diet and weight. Metabolic syndrome is a health condition inextricably linked to being overweight. The document establishes a goal "to reduce the proportion of children and adolescents who are overweight or obese" [80 p. 19-13]. Healthy People 2010 address food and nutrient consumption in the following goals:

- Increase the proportion of persons aged 2 years and older who consume at least two daily servings of fruit.
- Increase the proportion of persons aged 2 years and older who consume at least three daily servings of vegetables with at least one-third being dark green or orange vegetables.
- Increase the proportion of persons aged 2 years and older who consume at least six daily servings of grain products, with at least three being whole grains.
- Increase the proportion of persons aged 2 years and older who consume less than 10 percent of calories from saturated fat.
- Increase the proportion of persons aged 2 years and older who consume no more than 30 percent of calories from the total fat.

The Institute of Medicine (IOM) first introduced the report, "Preventing Childhood Obesity: Health in Balance" in 2005. [81] The IOM established the Standing Committee on Childhood Obesity Prevention in 2008 to address national policy issues specific to childhood obesity and guide the educational programming and research agenda for dissemination of information on prevention and treatment of childhood obesity in the United States. In the last decade, several programs have been implemented to support meeting health and nutrition goals for children and adolescents.

Team Nutrition and Healthier US Schools

The US Department of Agriculture (USDA) Food and Nutrition Service (FNS) developed the program Team Nutrition[82]. Team Nutrition is a child nutrition program that provides technical assistance and training to food service personnel, teachers, and caregivers. There are many resources to support the program ranging from classroom lesson plans on nutrition and physical activity to cookbooks and recipes that are healthy and fun to make.

Team Nutrition offers the opportunity for schools to enroll to become a Team Nutrition School that provides nutritional education to students; offers structures for the physical activity time for students; offers reimbursable lunches that demonstrate healthy menu planning that follow the practices and principles of the Dietary Guidelines of Americans and meet the USDA nutrition standards.

The FNS would like all schools to become involved in improving the nutrition of children and adolescents and achieving the goals for being recognized as a bronze, silver, or gold of *HealthierUS* Schools

Healthy dietary lifestyle and decision-making as well as daily physical activity behavior patterns should be introduced and reinforced beginning in early childhood and continued throughout adolescence.

The FNS Team Nutrition program goals are in alignment with the IOM Food and Nutrition report issued in 2007, "Nutrition Standards for Foods in Schools: Leading the Way to a Healthier Youth"[83] The report recommends food in the schools should be restricted to nutritious foods that meet the 2005 Dietary Guidelines for Americans.

School Health Screening Programs

School health screening program have been implemented to monitor anthropometric measurements—height, weight, BMI [84] . Arkansas, California, Delaware, Florida, Illinois, Kansas, Maine, Minnesota, Missouri, New York, Pennsylvania, Tennessee and West Virginia include states that legislate the use of a BMI health screening and parental notification as a means of monitoring the health of children specific to weight.

In an innovative school-based intervention program entitled: "Wellness, Academics, and You", Spiegel & Foulk [85]. investigated the BMI, consumption of fruits and vegetables, and physical activity of 1013 fourth and fifth grade students from 69 different classes in four states. The results of the study demonstrated that the BMI improved in the intervention group; consumption of fruits and vegetables increased in the intervention group; and physical activity also increased in the intervention group. The authors concluded that school-based programs may prove beneficial for reduction of overweight and obesity in children and adolescents.

Nutrition and Fitness Education through Model Curricula

Innovative education about health, nutrition, and fitness has been developed and implemented to address the concern of childhood obesity and the rise in diabetes mellitus in school age children.

PATHWAYS to Health Program

The PATHWAYS to Health Program[86] was an innovative study funded by the National Heart, Lung, and Blood Institute of the National Institutes of Health in 1993 in response to the rise in the number of American Indians who were overweight. The program was intended to provide the basis for a primary prevention model in the area of obesity and obesity related diseases within American Indian children. The study targeted young elementary school children before they formed their life-long habits. The PATHWAY program applies social learning theory to the acquisition of new behaviors such as the need to increase physical activity and make healthy eating choices.

The PATHWAY curriculum [86] is tailored for 3rd, 4th, and 5th graders. Children are provided with school-based lessons on content specific to food and nutrition science and the importance of physical activity. The curriculum also offers lessons in social learning theory facets such as self efficacy, changing behavior, mentoring, and peer support. The PATHWAY curriculum educates young American Indian children about developing a healthy life style through inclusion of learning that is personal, experiential, behavioral, and environmental. The results of the study demonstrated that the students were able to change and develop positive attitudes towards self-regulation of food choices and television viewing time duration.

Cherokee Choices/REACH

Cherokee Choices[87], a diabetes and obesity prevention program for American Indians, was introduced in 2000 and funded through the CDC program, "Racial and Ethnic Approaches to Community Health (REACH). The target population was Cherokee Indians living in North Carolina. The Cherokee Indians living in North Carolina were reported to have higher rates of type 2 diabetes and obesity than the North Carolina population in general and in the United States at large. One significant aspect of the Cherokee Choices/REACH program was providing health education to elementary (K-6) school children through a structured mentoring program. The mentors were hired to support the students as the school worked to change the health, nutrition, and fitness behaviors of 600 elementary school students. The mentors were included in the classrooms, recess, lunch period, and an afterschool program. The Cherokee Choices program was directed at making changes in the school health culture that improved the nutritional habits of the students and increased the physical activities.

Healthy Buddies

Healthy Buddies[88] is a health promotion program targeted at elementary school children in Canada. The project paired young children in Kindergarten to third grade with older children in the fourth to seventh grade. The project wanted to innovate a peer-led obesity and eating prevention program through developing a buddy system. Older students assumed the role of teachers for the younger students. In the student-led curriculum, the lessons provided to the students included healthy nutrition, the value of physical activity, and healthy body image.

The results of the study demonstrated that compared to the control group students, the younger and older intervention group students developed an increase in healthy living knowledge, attitudes, and behaviors. The students in the intervention group also had less weight gain and less increase in BMI and blood pressure. The Healthy Buddy program demonstrated that the older and younger students who participated in the student-led education curriculum each benefited from the program.

SUMMARY

Obesity in the United States is of epidemic proportions. The number of children and adolescents who are overweight and have Type 2 diabetes mellitus continues to rise. The metabolic syndrome and its long term health risks including cardiovascular disease, Type 2 diabetes mellitus, hypertension, nonalcoholic fatty liver disease, and PCOS are closely associated with obesity. A number of creative and effective projects and programs providing interventions for children and adolescents has been developed and are available with the focus on lifestyle modification which is fundamental to preventing and treating childhood obesity, metabolic syndrome, and the long term health consequences of these conditions. Establishing and maintaining healthy lifestyles in children especially related to diet and exercise is the best approach to preventing chronic health conditions in adults associated with obesity.

REFERENCES

[1] Cruz, ML; Shaiba, GQ; Weingensberg, MJ; Spruijt-Metz, D; Ball, G; Goran, MI. Pediatric Obesity and Insulin Resistance: Chronic Disease Risk and Implications for Treatment and Prevention Beyond Body Weight Modification. *Annu Rev Nutr*. 2005, 25, 435-468.

[2] De Ferranti, SD; Osganian, SK. Epidemiology of paediatric metabolic syndrome and type 2 diabetes mellitus. *Diabetes Vas Dis Res*., 2007, 4, 285-296.

[3] Rodriguez-Moran, M; Salazar-Vazquez, B; Violante, R; Guerrero-Romero, F. Metabolic Syndrome Among Children and Adolescents Aged 10-18 years. *Diabetes* 2004, 27, 2516-2527.

[4] Reaven,, GM. Role of insulin resistance in human disease. *Diabetes* 1988, 37, 1595-1607

[5] Reaven, GM. Hypertriglyceridemia:the central feature of syndrome X. *Cardiovasc Risk Factors,* 1996, 6, 29-35.

[6] Reaven, GM. Diet and Syndrome X. *Curr Atheroscler Rep*. 2000, 2, 503-507.

[7] Bonow, RO. Primary Prevention of Cardiovascular Disease. *Circulation,* 2002, 106, 31-40.

[8] Kim, SH; Reaven, GM. Insulin Resistance and Hyperinsulinemia-you can't have one without the other. *Diabetes,* 2008, 31, 1433-1438.

[9] De Ferranti, SD; Gauvreau, K; Ludwig, DS; Neufeld, EJ; Newburger, JW; Rifai, N. Prevalence of Metabolic Syndrome in American Adolescents: Findings from the Third National Health and Nutrition Examination Survey. *Circulation* 2004;110:2494-2497.

[10] Alberti, KG; Zimmet, PZ. Definition, diagnosis, and classification of diabetes mellitus and its complications. Part 1. Diagnosis and classification of diabetes mellitus provisional report of WHO consultation. *Diabetes Med*., 1998, 15, 539-553.

[11] Grundy, SM; Cleeman, C; Merz, NB; Brewer, HB., et al. Implications of Recent Clinical Trials for the National Cholesterol Education Program Adult Treatment Panel III Guidelines. *Circulation,* 2004, 110, 227-239.

[12] Lorenzo, C; Okoloise, M; Williams, K; Stein, MP; Haffner, SM. The Metabolic Syndrome as Predictor of Type 2 Diabetes—The San Antonio Health Study. *Diabetes Care,* 2003, 26, 3153-3159.

[13] Duncan, GE; Li SM; Zhou XH. Prevalence and Trends of Metabolic Syndrome Phenotype Among U.S. Adolescents, 1999-2000. *Diabetes Care,* 2004, 27, 2438-2443.

[14] Http://www.cdc.gov/nchs. Accessed on March 12, 2009.

[15] Hirschler V; Maccallini G; Calcagno M; Aranda C; Jadzinsky M. Waist circumference identifies primary school children with metabolic syndrome abnormalities. ; *Diabetes Technology & Therapeutics*, 2007; 9: 149-157.

[16] Sorof, JM; Lai, D; Turner, J; Poffenbarger, T; Portman, RJ. Overweight, Ethnicity, and the Prevalence of Hypertension in School-Aged Children. *Pediatrics,* 2004, 113, 475-482.

[17] The Endocrine Society. Prevention and Treatment of Pediatric Obesity: An Endocrine Society Clinical Practice Guideline Based on Expert Opinion. *J. Clin Endo Met.,* 2008, 93, 4576-4599.

[18] Camhi, SM; Kuo, J; Young, DR. Identifying Adolescent Metabolic Syndrome Using Body Mass Index and Waist Circumference. *Prev Chronic Dis*. 2008, 5(4). http://www.cdcc.gov/pcd/issues/2008/0ct/07_0170.htm. Accessed on January 19, 2009.

[19] National High Blood Pressure Education Program Working Group on High Blood Pressure in Children and Adolescents. The Fourth Report on the Diagnosis, Evaluation, and Treatment of High Blood Pressure in Children and Adolescents. *Pediatrics,* 2004, 114, 555-576.

[20] Angulo, P. Obesity and Nonalcoholic Fatty Liver Disease. *Nutrition Reviews,* 2007, 11, S57-S-63

[21] Morrison, JA; Friedman, LA; Gray-McGuire, C. Metabolic syndrome in childhood predicts adult cardiovascular disease 25 years later: the Princeton Lipids Research Follow-up Study. *Pediatrics,* 2007, 120, 340-345.

[22] Paradis, G; Lamber, MO; Loughlin, J; Lavallee, C., et al. Blood Pressure and Adiposity in Children and Adolescents. *Circulation,* 2005, 143, 1832-1838.

[23] Writing Group for SEARCH for Diabetes in Youth Study Group, Dabelea D, Bell RA, D'Agostino RB, et al. Incidence of diabetes in youth in the United States. *JAMA,* 2007, 297, 2716-2724.

[24] Rodriguez, BL; Fujimoto, WY; Mayer-Davis, EJ., et al. Prevalence of Cardiovascular Disease Risk Factors in U.S. Children and Adolescents With Diabetes-The SEARCH for Diabetes in Youth Study *Diabetes Care,* 2006, 29, 1891-1896.

[25] Adams, LA; Angulo, P. Recent concepts in non-alcoholic fatty liver disease. *Diabet Med.*, 2005, 22, 1129-1133.

[26] Stein, IF; Leventhal, ML. Amenorrhea associated with bilateral polycystic ovaries. *Am J Obstet Gynecol.,* 1935, 29, 181-191.

[27] Azziz, R; Marin, C; Hoq, L., et al. Health care-related economic burden of the polycystic ovary syndrome during the reproductive life span. *J Clin Endocrinol Metab.,* 2005, 90, 4650-4658.

[28] Goodarzi, MO; Azziz, R. Diagnosis, epidemiology, and genetics of the polycystic ovary syndrome. *Best Pract. Res Clin Endocrinol Metab*., 2006, 20, 193-205.

[29] Ehrmann, DA. Polycystic ovary syndrome. *NEJM*., 2005, 352, 1223-1237.

[30] Ibanez, L; Potau, N; Virdis, R., et al. Postpubertal outcome in girls diagnosed of premature pubarche during childhood: increased frequency of functional ovarian hyperandrogenism. *J Clin Endocrinol Metab*., 1993, 76, 1599-1603.

[31] Ibanez, L; Potau, N; Zampoll, M., et al. Hyperinsulinemia and decreased insulin-like growth factor-binding protein 1 are common features in prepubertal and pubertal girls with a history of premature pubarche. *J Clin Endocrnol Metab.,* 1997, 21, 2283-2288.

[32] Ibanez, L; Dimartino-Nardi, J; Potau., et al. Premature adrenarche- normal variant or forerunner of adult disease? *Endocr Rev.*, 2000, 21; 671-696.

[33] Abbott, DH; Dumesic, DA; Franks, F. Developmental origin of polycystic ovary syndrome-a hypothesis. *J Endocrinol.*, 2002, 174, 1-5.

[34] Franks, S; McCarthy, MI; Hardy, K. Development of polycystic ovary syndrome: involvement of genetic and environmental factors. *Int J Androl.,* 2006, 29, 278-85, discussion 286-290.

[35] Meas, T; Chevenne, D; Thibaud, E., et al. Endocrine consequences of premature pubarche in post-pubertal Caucasian girls. *Clin Endocrinol (Oxf).* 2002, 57, 101-106.

[36] Dimartino-Nardi, J. Premature adrenarche: findings in prepubertal African-American and Caribbean-Hispanic girls. *Acta Paediatr Suppl.*, 1999, 88, 67-72.

[37] Vuguin, P; Linder, B; Rosenfeld, RG., et al. The roles of insulin sensitivity, insulin-like growth factor I (IGF I), and IGF-binding-protein-1 and-3 in the hypoandrogenism of African-American and Caribbean Hispanic girls with premature adrenarche. *J Clin Endocr Metab.*, 1999, 84, 2037-2042.

[38] Ibanez, L; Potau, N; Francois, I., et al. Precocious pubarche, hyperinsulinism, and ovarian hyperandrogenism in girls: relation to reduced fetal growth. *J Clin Endocrinol Metab.*, 1998, 83, 3558-3562.

[39] Wiksten-Almstromer, M; Hirschberg, AL; Hagenfeldt, K. Menstrual disorders and associated factors among adolescent girls visiting a youth clinic. *Acta Obstet Gynecol Scand.*, 2007, 86, 65-72.

[40] Coviello, AD; Legro, RS; Dunaif, A. Adolescent girls with polycystic ovary syndrome have an increased risk of metabolic syndrome associated with increasing androgen levels independent of obesity and insulin resistance. *J Clin Endocrinol Metab.*, 2006, 91, 393-395.

[41] Zawadski, JK; Dunaif, A. Diagnostic criteria for polycystic ovary syndrome: towards a rational approach. In: Dunaif A, Givens JR, Haseltine FP, et al. editors. Polycystic ovary syndrome. Cambridge, *Blackwell Scientific Publications*, 1992, pp. 377-384.

[42] Rotterdam ESHRE/ASRM Sponsored PCOS Consensus Workshop Group. Revised 2003 consensus on diagnostic criteria and long term health risks related to poly cystic ovary syndrome. *Fertil Steril.*, 2004, 81, 19-25.

[43] Azziz, R; Carmina, E; Dewailly, D., et al. Position Statement: Criteria for defining polycystic ovary syndrome as a predominant hyperandogenic syndrome: An Androgen Excess Society Guideline. *J Clin Endocrinol Metab.,* 2006, 91, 4237-4245.

[44] Franks, S; Gharani, N; Waterworth, D., et al. The genetic basis of polycystic ovary syndrome. *Hum Reprod.*, 1997, 12, 2641-2648.

[45] Legro, RS; Driscoll, D; Strauss III, JF., et al. Evidence for a genetic basis for hyperandrogenemia in polycystic ovary syndrome. *Proc Natl Acad Sci,* USA, 1998, 95, 14956-14960.

[46] Vink, JM; Sanrzadeh, S; Lambalk, CB., et al. Heritability of polycystic ovary syndrome (PCOS) in a Dutch twin-family study. *J Clin Endocrinol Metab.*, 2006, 91, 2100-2104.

[47] Legro, RS; Bentley-Lewis, R; Driscoll, D., et al. Insulin resistance in the sisters of women with polycystic ovary syndrome: association with hyperandrogenemia rather than menstrual irregularity. *J Clin Endocrinol Metab.,* 2002, 87, 2128-2133.

[48] Salmi, DJ; Zisser, HC; Jovanovic, L. Screening for and treatment of polycystic ovary syndrome in teenagers. *Exp Biol Med.*, 2004, 229, 369-377.

[49] Huber-Buchholz, MM; Carey, DG; Norman, RJ. Restoration of reproductive potential by lifestyle modification in obese polycystic ovary syndrome: role of insulin sensitivity and luteinizing hormone. *J Clin Endocrinol Metab.*, 1999, 84, 1470-1474.

[50] Hoeger, KM; Kochman, L; Wixom, N., et al. A randomized, 48 week, placebo-controlled trial of intensive lifestyle modification and/or metformin therapy in overweight women with polycystic ovary syndrome: a pilot study. *Fertil Steril.*, 2004, 82, 421-429.

[51] Wabitsch, M; Hauner, H; Heinze, E., et al. Body fat distribution and steroid hormone concentrations in obese adolescent girls before and after weight reduction. *J Clin Endocrinol Metab.*, 1995, 80, 3469-3475.

[52] Reinehr, T., De Sousa, G; Roth, CL., et al. Androgens before and after weight loss in children. *J Clin Endocrinol Metab.*, 2005, 90, 5588-5595.

[53] Franks, S. Polycystic ovary syndrome. *NEJM.*, 1995, 333, 853-861.

[54] Dunaif, A. Insulin resistance and the polycystic ovary syndrome: mechanism and implications for pathogenesis. *Endocr Rev.*, 1997, 18, 774-800.

[55] Kiddy, DS; Sharp, PS; White, DM., et al. Differences between clinical and endocrine features between obese and non-obese subjects with polycystic ovary syndrome: an analysis of 263 consecutive cases. *Clin Endocr (Oxf.),* 1990, 32, 213-220.

[56] Holte, J; Bergh, T; Berne, T., et al. Serum lipoprotein lipid profile in women with the polycystic ovary syndrome: relation to anthropometric, endocrine and metabolic variables. *Clin Endocr (Oxf.).,* 1194, 41, 463-471.

[57] Franks, S. Polycystic ovary syndrome: a changing perspective. *Clin Endocr (Oxf.).* 1989, 31, 87-120.

[58] Legro, RS. The genetics of obesity: lessons for polycystic ovary syndrome. *Ann N Y Acad Sci.*, 2000, 900, 193-202.

[59] Azziz, R. Androgen excess in women: experience with over 1000 consecutive patients. *J Clin Endocrinol Metab.*, 2004, 89, 453-462.

[60] Lewy, VD; Danadian, K; Witchel; SF., et al. Early metabolic abnormalities in adolescent girls with polycystic ovarian syndrome. *J Pediatr.*, 2001, 138, 38-44.

[61] Silfen, ME; Denburg, MR; Manibo, AM., et al. Early endocrine, metabolic and sonographic characteristics if polycystic ovary syndrome (PCOS): Comparison between obese and non-obese adolescents. *J Clin Endocrinol Metab.,* 2003, 88, 4682-4688.

[62] Legro, RS. Detection of insulin resistance and its treatment in adolescents with polycystic ovary syndrome. *J Pediatr Endocrinol Metab.,* 2002, 15 (suppl 5), 1367-1378.

[63] American Diabetes Association. Type 2 diabetes in children and adolescents. *Pediatrics*, 2000, 105(3 pt 1), 671-680.

[64] Palmert, MR; Gordon, CM; Kartashov, AI., et al. Screening for abnormal glucose tolerance in adolescents with polycystic ovary syndrome. *J Clin Endocrinol Metab.,* 2002, 87, 1017-1023.

[65] Apridonidze, T; Essah, PA; Iuorno, MJ., et al. Prevalence and characteristics of the metabolic syndrome in women with polycystic ovary syndrome. *J Clin Endocrinol Metab.,* 2005, 90, 1929-1935.

[66] Ford, ES; Giles, WH; Dietz, WH. Prevalence of the metabolic syndrome among US adults: Findings from the third National Health and Nutrition Survey. *JAMA.*, 2002, 287, 356-359.

[67] Talbott, EO; Guzick, DS; Sutton-Tyrrell, K., et al. Evidence for association between polycystic ovary syndrome and premature carotid atherosclerosis in middle-aged women. *Arterioscler Thromb Vasc Biol.* 2000, 20, 2414-2421.

[68] Orio, F; Jr, Palomba, S; Cascella, T., et al. Early impairment of endothelial structure and function in young normal weight womenwith polycystic ovary syndrome. *J Clin Endocrinol Metab.*, 2004, 89, 4588-4593.

[69] Vryonidou, A; Papatheodorou, A; Tavridou, A., et al. Association of hyperandrogenemic and metabolic phenotype with carotid intima-media thickness in young women with polycystic ovary syndrome. *J Clin Endocrinol Metab.,* 2005, 90, 2740-2746.

[70] Ehrmann, DA; Barnes, RB; Rosenfield, RL., et al. Prevalence of impaired glucose tolerance and diabetes in women with polycystic ovary syndrome. *Diabetes Care.*, 1999, 22, 141-146.

[71] Legro, RS; Kunselman, AR; Dodson, WC., et al. Prevalence and predictors of risk for type 2 diabetes mellitus and impaired glucose tolerance in polycystic ovary syndrome: a prospective controlled study in 254 affected women. *J Clin Endorinol Metab.*, 1999, 84, 165-169.

[72] Legro, RS; Gnatuk, CL; Kunselman, AR., et al. Changes in glucose tolerance over time in women with polycystic ovary syndrome: a controlled study. *J Clin Endocrinol Metab.*, 2005, 90, 3236-3242.

[73] Eckel, RH; Grundy, SM; Zimmet, PZ. The metabolic syndrome. *Lancet.* 2005, 365, 1415-1428.

[74] Schmeler, KM; Soliman, PT; Sun, CC., et al. Endometrial cancer in young, normal weight women. *Gynecologic oncology.* 2005, 99, 388-392.

[75] Kurman, RJ; Kaminski, PF; Norris, HJ. The behavior of endometrial hyperplasia. A long-term study of untreated hyperplasia in 170 patients. *Cancer.* 1985, 56, 403-412.

[76] Soliman, PT, Oh, JC; Schmeler, KM., et al. Risk factors for young premenopausal women with endometrial cancer. *Obstet Gynecol.* 2005, 105, 575-580.

[77] Froeschle, JG; Castillo, Y; Mayorga, MG., et al. Counseling techniques for adolescent females with polycystic ovary syndrome. *J Prof Counsel: Pract Theo and Res.,* 2008, 36, 17-29

[78] Rofey, DL; Szigethy, EM; Noll, RB., et al. Cognitive-behavioral therapy for physical and emotional disturbances in adolescents with polycystic ovary syndrome: a pilot study. *J pediatric Psychol.*, 2008, June 21, pp. 1-8.

[79] Trent, ME; Rich, M; Austin, SB., et al. Quality of life in adolescent girls with polycystic ovary syndrome. *Arch Pediatr Adolesc Med.*, 2002, 156, 556-560.

[80] U. S. Department of Health and Human Services. *Healthy People 2010*. 2nd ed. *With Understanding and Improving Health and Objectives and Objectives for Improving Health*. 2 vols. Washington, D.C.: U.S. Government Printing Office, 2000.

[81] Jeffrey, P. Koplan, Catharyn T. Liverman, and Vivica A. Kraak, Editors, Committee on Prevention of Obesity in Children and Youth. *Preventing Childhood Obesity: Health in the Balance* . Washington, D.C.: National Academies Press, 2005.

[82] USDA Team Nutrition: *Guidelines for training food service professionals to achieve healthy school meals.* Alexandria, VA: U.S. Dept. of Agriculture, Food and Consumer Service, 1995.

[83] McGinnis, JM; Gootman, JA; Kraak, VI., eds. *Food marketing to children and youth: threat or opportunity?* Washington, D.C.: National Academies Press, 2006.

[84] Kubik, MY; Story, M; Rieland, G. Developing School-Based BMI Screening and Parent Notification Programs: Findings From Focus Groups With Parents of Elementary School Students. *J. Health Education and Behavior,* 2007, 34, 622-633.

[85] Spiegel, SA; Foulk, D. Reducing Overweight through a Multidisciplinary School-based Intervention. *Obesity,* 2006, 14, 88-96.

[86] Riggs, NR; Sakuma, KK; Pentz, MA. Preventing Risk for Obesity by Promoting Self-Regulation and Decision-Making Skills: Pilot Results from the PATHWAYS to Health Program (PATHWAYS). *Eval Rev*., 2007, 31, 287-310.

[87] Bachar, JJ; Lefler, LJ; Reed, L; McCoy, T., et al. *Prev Chronic Dis*. 2005; 3(3).http://www.cdc.gov/pcd/issues/2006/jul05_0221 htm. Accessed on February 1, 2009.

[88] Stock, S; Miranda, C; Evans, S; Plessis, S., et al. Healthy Buddies: A Novel, Peer-Led Health Promotion Program for Prevention of Obesity and Eating Disorders in Children in Elementary School. *Pediatrics,* 2007, 120, 1059-1068.

In: Nutritional Education
Editor: Ida R. Laidyth

ISBN: 978-1-60876-078-7

Chapter 6

INFORMATION TECHNOLOGY IN TERTIARY LEVEL NUTRITION EDUCATION

A. Wise
The Robert Gordon University, St Andrew St, Aberdeen, Scotland

ABSTRACT

The paper reviews methods for enhancing learning at tertiary level by using information technology, including published examples relevant to nutrition education of adults in other contexts. Teaching may include animations that enhance understanding and personal response systems that provide immediate feedback about student comprehension. Tutorials, practical classes and self-study materials can incorporate a wide range of computer programs. These have been used for many years to permit students to analyse their own diets, which is known to provide useful feedback to enable changes to be made. Students learn from exercises in which they have to improve diets and they can become more familiar with food composition using computer-generated bar charts in a quiz format. Programs can integrate energy expenditure with different levels of activity to energy intake with different diets. Students may learn how vitamins are involved in metabolism by exploring pathways using an interactive program. Student research projects can be enhanced by using a program that helps them write a protocol and the output of statistical programs can be interpreted by a program that reads the screen and explains what it means. Computers can be used as vehicles for simulations of practical situations such as client interviews and they can provide discussion forums for students on placement. Whilst revising before assessments, students may benefit from a variety of testing programs; for example crossword puzzles test their knowledge in an enjoyable way and construction of sentences using words from a list tests their understanding of concepts.

INTRODUCTION

Nutrition is taught at different levels to a wide range of students at tertiary level. In the UK alone, the University and College Admissions' Service listed approximately 300 awards in nutrition, a substantial increase in provision since the previous review in 1991 that reported only 19 awards in nutrition (Nutrition Society, 2005). Many modular programmes often combined nutrition with a diverse range of science and other subjects. In 2000, there were 2,065 nutrition graduates of all kinds. Over a 15-year period, there was a 2.7 fold increase in the number of universities in the UK that offered taught postgraduate courses leading to the award of an MSc in nutrition: 19 in 2005, compared with 7 in 1989. There is thus evidence of an extraordinary increase in graduate provision of nutrition training. Nutrition is also required for a wide range of other health-related and food-related disciplines such as medicine, dentistry, pharmacy, nursing and catering. Since children need to be taught some nutrition, it is needed to some degree in training teachers.

Many lecturing staff in tertiary level education find that much of their time is taken up with research and hence development of teaching methods may not get the attention it deserves (Higher Education Academy, 2009). Whilst nutritionists were early adopters of computers to speed up calculation of dietary analyses, they have not generally taken such a great interest in how information technology can be used to enhance their teaching. There are not a great number of publications in this area, but this paper attempts to review some developments and use my experience in an attempt to stimulate nutrition lecturers to evaluate them more fully in future.

ENHANCING LECTURES

Perhaps the most obvious place for Information Technology in the classroom is presentation software such as PowerPoint. In the past, lecturers used the blackboard, then developed the use of overhead projection of acetates or slides, but now PowerPoint has become routine for many. Frey & Birnbaum (2002) reviewed the literature and found one study that showed students could achieve better grades when PowerPoint was used in lectures, and then further investigated students' ideas of this technology. The majority of students had positive perceptions: 69% agreed that PowerPoint presentations held their attention and 79% perceived their lecturers who used PowerPoint were more organised during lectures. Students particularly valued printing PowerPoint slides as handouts and 91% thought they helped them to study, in particular with reference to emphasis on key points.

The use of PowerPoint to emphasise the key points during a lecture may seem so mainstream now that it hardly deserves this attention, but there are many issues in nutrition that are complex and can benefit from the use of animations that are easy to achieve in PowerPoint and similar software. Figure 1 illustrates a slide the author uses to explain how blocking can be used to design a study comparing additional Zn to a control diet by choosing subjects that match in starting weight. During the lecture, the figures with similar weights move on a mouse click to their positions in each block using a custom path.

Flash videos are even more useful when trying to explain complex material, especially metabolic pathways or control of metabolism. For example, a Flash video was used successfully to illustrate part of a figure explaining how transcription factors are involved in the control of macronutrient metabolism (Wise, 2008a). In this case, glucagon is shown interacting with its receptor, causing production of cyclic AMP and the phosphorylated transcription factor CREBP is shown promoting production of PGC-1, which will later move to a second DNA sequence in the video to enhance the promoting effects of HNF-4 in the transcription of genes for enzymes involved in gluconeogenesis. Since this is such a complex series of events, it is very difficult to explain without graphical support. During the lecture, the video is played in steps and the previous steps can be repeated on request until the students feel that they have understood the mechanism. The video can be made available for students to study later when they wish.

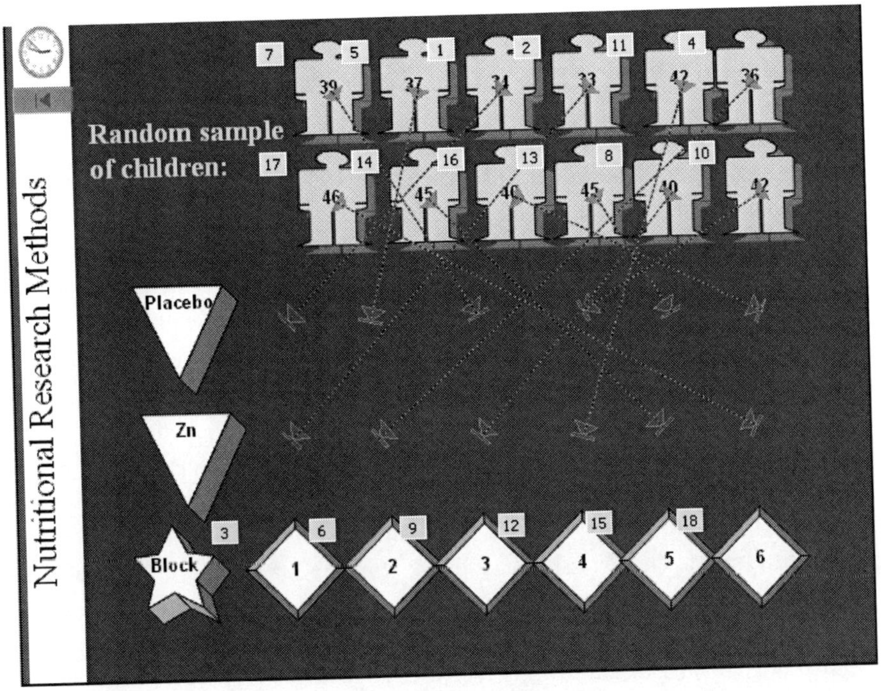

Figure 1. Enhancement of lectures using animation in PowerPoint

Another technology that has been developing considerably lately is known by several different names, for example the personal response system (eInstruction, 2009). Using radio receivers and transmitters in clickers, students can interact with the lecturer in large numbers during a lecture and provide instant feedback to questions, which can be linked to a PowerPoint presentation. The manufacturer claims that this method allows you to immediately chart student responses, increase class participation, identify areas where students need more help and encourage group and peer learning.

Gachago (2008) has undertaken detailed research into the use of this system by 31 science lecturers at the University of Edinburgh. Several lecturers used clickers in innovative ways, such as encouraging students to discuss with their peers before voting (n=10). Some lecturers also ask students to revote on questions (n=13), after having explained a question in more detail or allowing students to discuss with their peers. Three lecturers used confidence levels, which show how confident students are when selecting a voting option. Confidence levels in conjunction with re-voting is said to give some interesting insights into students' increasing level of confidence in their own knowledge and understanding of a concept. The lecturers were asked to rank by importance several reasons for using clickers and with a maximum possible score of 500 they considered that the system: increases interaction between lecturers and students (score=456); provides feedback on students' understanding of content (score=437); reveals common misconceptions amongst students (score=415) and helps students understand difficult concepts better (score=406).

SELF-STUDY PROGRAMS

Underpinning Subjects

Tutorials, practical classes and self-study materials can incorporate a wide range of computer programs. One of the underpinning elements to a nutrition course is biochemistry and in particular they need to understand metabolic pathways involved in processing and use of nutrients. Nicholson (2008) has produced a series of Flash videos that show how the molecules glide in and out of enzymes and the reactions are well explained step by step at http://www.iubmb-nicholson.org/animaps.html. The well-known wall chart produced by Roche Applied Science (2009) can be accessed online and users can search for a key word or click on the map itself to see part of it. GenomeNet (2002) provides overview diagrams illustrating sections of metabolism with hotspots that can be clicked to provide detailed information on the enzymes including amino acid and base sequences. These resources are extremely valuable for students who are studying biochemistry in depth, but they are arguably too complex and information intensive for many nutrition students. The metabolic pathways program was designed to help nutrition students learn about the main metabolic pathways, and in particular the ways in which vitamins are used in metabolism (Wise, 2002a). The approach to program design was to make it as interactive as possible to enhance exploration and understanding of interrelationships between substances via the inclusion of many hotspots on the screen for navigation and provision of relevant information.

The top frame contains a menu, which includes links to a ‘contents’ page or a popup map showing the outline of basic metabolic pathways (see Figure 2). There is a menu item that provides a list of vitamins that are required as coenzymes, for example choosing folate leads to a list of reactions requiring it, each of which can be clicked to show the pathway on the left of the screen. Clicking on the arrow between the two substrates generally shows the structures of the metabolites along with the name of the enzyme, and clicking on the coenzyme gives its structure and list of reactions requiring it. Since some metabolites also act as allosteric modifiers elsewhere in metabolism, this is indicated when appropriate so that the student is taken to the reaction to see what effect it has.

Research is an important aspect of nutrition so that students need to learn research design and statistical analysis. This is a notoriously difficult area to teach and for students to comprehend fully so if they can study using information technology and gain some insights doing so this is a very useful application for their learning. Although statistical programs are very powerful tools for statisticians, unfortunately they tend not to be very simple and the output may be difficult to interpret. Therefore, if students undertake a practical class in statistics applied to nutritional problems, they are continually asking what the information means, or they just look at it cursorily and do not understand but are too embarrassed to say so. In order to try to improve on this situation, a program was written by Wise (2003) that reads the screen of the statistical program Minitab and interprets the figures on it for the student (see Figure 3). This was not as highly rated as some of the other support material for this subject, but it has been improved since then and seems to be helpful to students since they are observed to use it frequently and they ask fewer simple questions during practical classes.

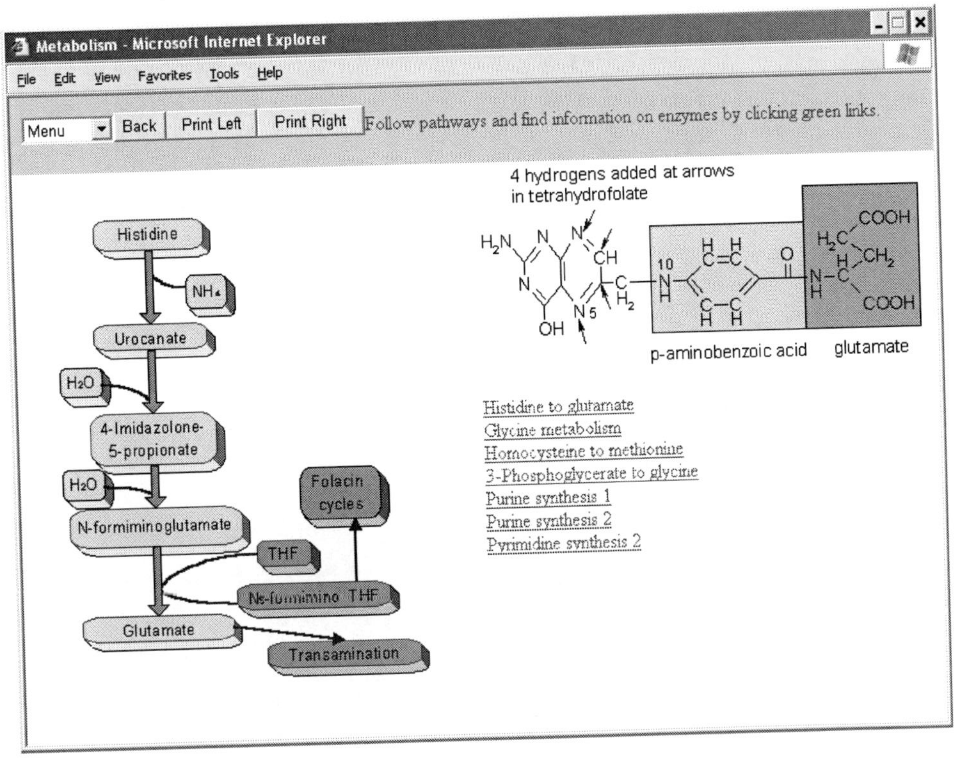

Figure 2. Metabolic pathways program

Research methods do not only contain statistical tests, but include a wide range of material to enable them to comprehend the scientific literature and undertake research: sampling, type I and type II errors, validity, confounding, definition of units, levels and factors, and a host of different types of bias and ways to attempt to avoid them (Heath, 1995; Huck & Cormier, 1996). It is particularly important that students should understand these concepts and apply them in their reading of the literature, so the examination includes simulated sentences from research papers with blank spaces to complete. A program was written that appears in a web page and 20 sentences are chosen at random from those that are similar to the ones in the examination. Each sentence has two spaces to be filled and the 40 missing words are arranged in alphabetical order on the left of the screen. When students think they have identified a missing word, they indicate it and the place in the sentence where they think it belongs. If they have correctly identified the missing word, the sentence is rewritten to include the word. It was generally agreed that the sentences could not easily be guessed by using grammatical rules and that the puzzle program had helped them to understand the material and prepare for the examination. Most (78%) students copied many of the sentences in the puzzle program onto paper for use in the open book examination and 69% agreed that the program was clearly laid out and easy to operate. When comparing this program with eight other types of support materials provided in the module, average scores (out of 10) were in decreasing order 8.28 for the mock examination, 8.09 for the handout and then 7.53 for the web-based puzzle program. It is interesting to note that students differed considerably in their opinion of the different support materials. For each of them, there was at least one student who rated it 0-2 and another who rated it 9-10. Thus it is important to provide a wide range of types of support material to cater for the individual learning styles of each student and it can not be expected that all will engage with methods involving information technology. This type of program in which students build sentences can also be used in a wide range of nutritional subjects where understanding of concepts needs to be built.

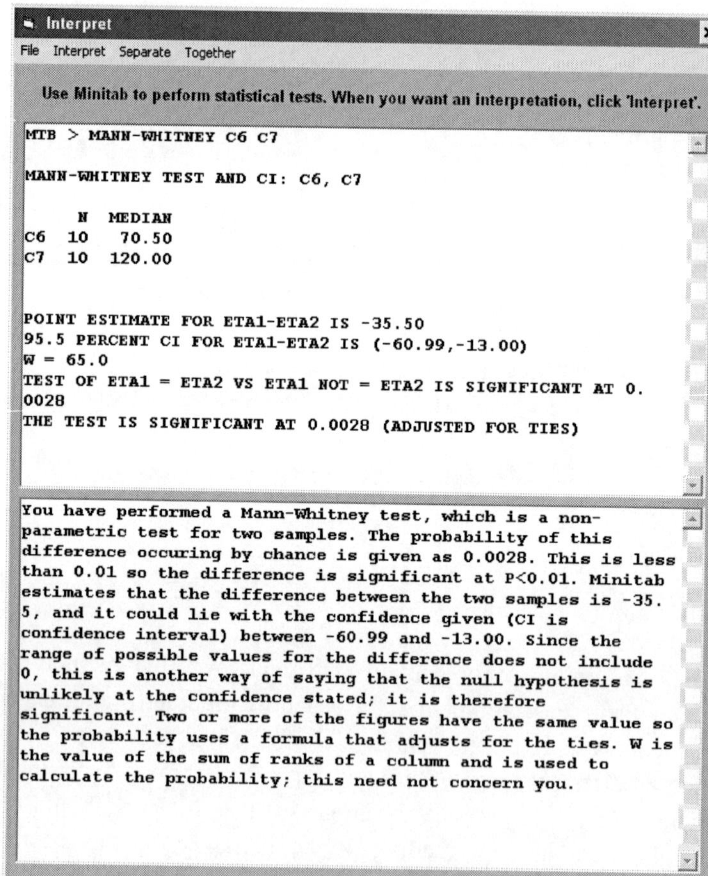

Figure 3. Inperpret Minitab program

Applied Nutritional Subjects

Programs have been used for many years to permit students to analyse their own diets, which is known to provide useful feedback to enable changes to be made (Kroeze et al. 2006). Although it may be argued that students only need to learn information to pass assessments, if they are to help others to change their diets it may be a good idea to be able to do this themselves first. Students also learn from exercises in which they have to improve diets because they have to search for foods that would be nutritionally more appropriate than those in the diet provided. An example of this concept is shown in Figure 4. Students were provided with a diet designed to be able to be considerably improved if they could find and apply 8 different nutritional messages to the client, for example to change from white to wholemeal bread. They can be assessed by what proportion of these messages they employ and the report they write about the changes they suggest. The main requirement to facilitate this type of educational experience is to provide students with a nutritional analysis program designed for education such as WinDiets (www.windiets.com; Wise, 2006; Wise, 2008b).

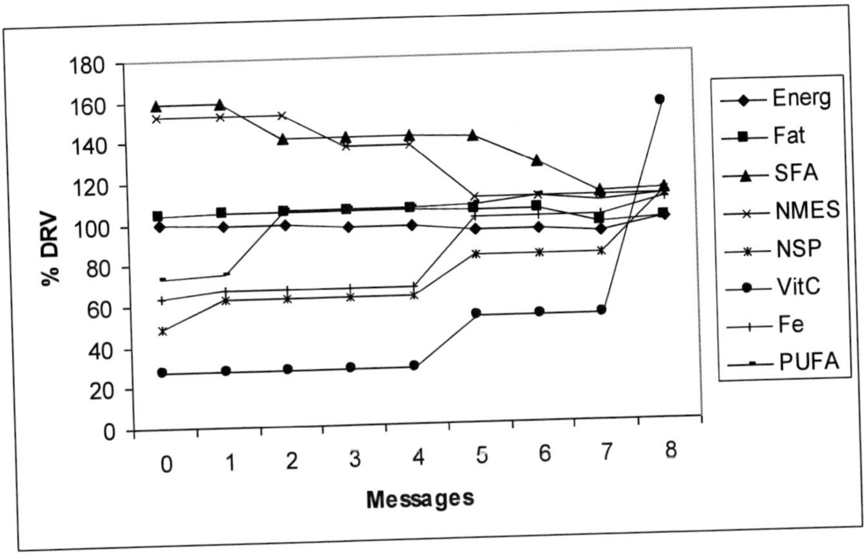

Figure 4. Exercise for students to improve a diet

The innovation in WinDiets that is particularly designed to help students choose appropriate foods is that the program is designed around a web-based window in which pictures and colours are used to provide information along with the expected dietary analyses in tables and graphs. It is important that students get an understanding of portion sizes of food so they can look at photographs of different weighed portions of a variety of foods in the program. This is facilitated by providing a list of foods that match search criteria, each with a background colour, the intensity of which relates to the amount of a chosen nutrient in the food. Students can preview the main nutrient content and information about portion weights of the foods on the screen by clicking those that appear in the list. A particularly novel feature of using colour intensity is a screen that permits students to compare two foods directly for energy content. Colour intensity is also employed to show visually what foods contribute most to the main nutrients in a meal (see Figure 5).

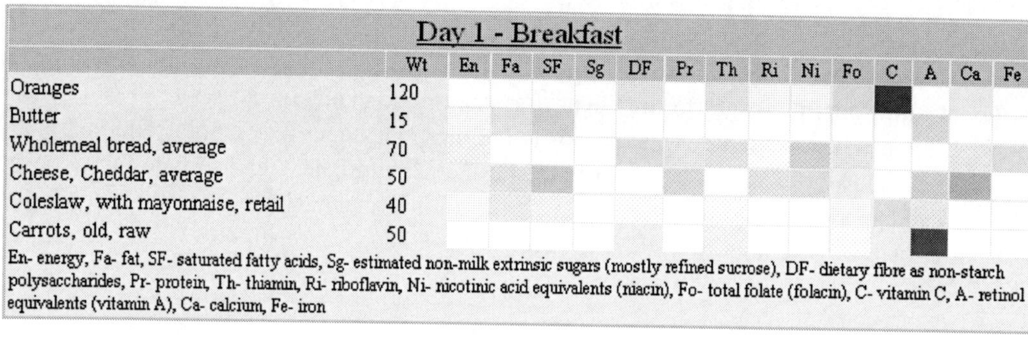

Figure 5. Composition of a meal illustrated using the intensity of colour

Another method that can be used to help students learn the main nutritional components in foods is a screen that presents a quiz of the composition of foods in which nutritional analyses are shown in bar charts compared to dietary reference values (Wise, 2002b). The quiz screen has been developed so that it contains a program that randomly presents a bar chart of an individual food and provides a list of 10 foods to choose from, including the one in the bar chart. After choosing a food from the list, students are shown the correct answer if they made a mistake and they are provided with a score that they can try to improve by choosing a higher proportion of correct foods. Students are unlikely to be able to buy this program, but many of them have computers at home and use them for study. Therefore, WinDiets permits the building of a quiz by selection of appropriate foods to include and export of the resultant quiz as an independent web page that can be put on the lecturer's web site for student use at home. Second stage students were shown the program in a tutorial and 16 of the students completed an anonymous questionnaire about their attitudes to the program. Most (n=15) found it user-friendly and agreed that they were more motivated to learn by having the score of their attempts than having no score (n=14). There was little agreement with the proposition that they would prefer to learn about nutritional composition from a book than a computer (n=1) and there was overwhelming disagreement (n=15) with a statement that 'food composition is such a simple subject that it does not deserve time in an Honours Nutrition course'.

Programs can integrate energy expenditure with different levels of activity to energy intake with different diets. These depend on the basal metabolic rate (BMR), which can be applied during sleep and the extent of physical activity during the day. The UK Government's publication on reference nutrient intakes suggests a method for calculating individual energy requirements based on BMR and activity (Department of Health, 1991). A simpler Internet version of the program showed how manipulating factors can alter energy balance (Wise & Cowie, 2005). It helped students to test out the effect of varying lifestyles on energy requirements and has been incorporated into WinDiets. The screen has a grid of numbers on the right. Each of these represents what a person is doing for a 5-minute period. There are 12 figures per hour and when a student enters the program, the data are all set at 1 to represent the physical activity ratio (PAR) of sleep. The student selects a time of rising by clicking the relevant part of the grid. The student can select from one of the eight PAR buttons on the left of the screen. This is entered into the grid and the student can continue clicking the buttons on the left of the screen and the data is entered into the grid until it is time to retire to bed again. The program was used in a practical class to introduce the way energy requirements depend on activity. Students were instructed to enter data typical of a sedentary person, and then discover how requirements alter as people lose or gain weight. They were told to alter the data to include a tennis match or other sports activity. It may be particularly surprising how little this may alter energy expenditure, especially if students are told to calculate what difference a single tennis match would make over a week. Having found the extra energy needed for exercise, students can calculate how much fat could be lost and how long it would take to achieve substantial weight loss assuming the energy value of tissue lost. Assuming 38 kJ/g for fat, the least weight that could be lost would be 26 g/MJ deficit, but since adipose tissue contains more than fat and other tissues are also lost during periods of negative energy balance, a higher value would be appropriate (Garrow, 1978). In the first few days, a high proportion of water is lost but after a few weeks of negative energy balance, losses of about 32 g/MJ could be predicted. Another exercise that was very revealing to students was to provide them with some confectionery that contains a nutritional label and calculate how long they would have to run before they have oxidised this energy-rich snack.

This tutorial has been improved by using screens in WinDiets that permit selection from about 600 different activities and outputs energy balance every hour during the day. Figure 6 illustrates part of the work involved in the tutorial. A subject is simply lying all day but eats three meals and is in energy balance at the end of the day. Then she takes some confectionary as a snack in the morning and is in positive balance over the day. Finally she plays an hour of tennis in the afternoon and is back almost in balance so the student can see that the confectionary requires an hour of tennis to oxidise it.

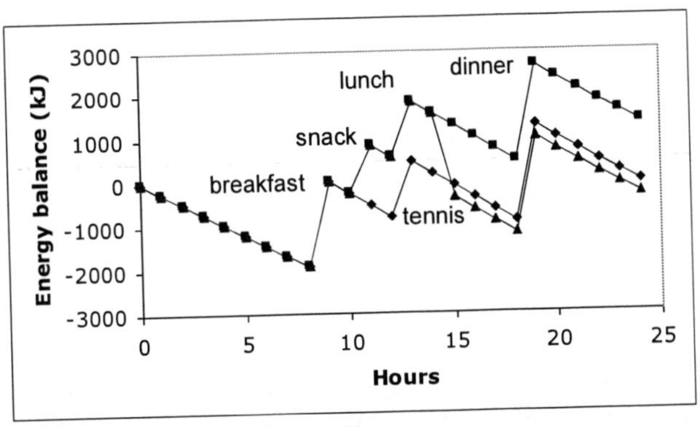

Figure 6. Graph of energy balance during the day to illustrate the importance of diet and activity

Students studying nutrition and dietetics may use specially written programs to help prepare them for the clinical environment (Herriot et al. 2004). The program facilitated learning how to take a diet history, to calculate nutrient intake and then use this information, together with an understanding of an individual's medical and social history, to advise on dietary change. The majority of students believed the program was a good method for preparing them for placement and particularly highly rated it for the dietetic interview, dietitians record card, medical notes and doctor's referral letters.

Litchfield et al. (2002) also claimed that online education of dietitians improved their performance in certain aspects of their competence. Turner et al. (2000) investigated the use of two different computer programs so that use of a computer was not a confounding factor, but this means that it can not be shown that either was better than another form of education.

They produced a care planning simulation system with 3 patient cases and students accessed patient information and developed a dietetic care plan. This was compared to a program that covered data collection, interpretation and care plan development in a drill and practice format. Performance on placement was then rated by dietitians and it was found that those who learned through the simulation program improved their performance faster than the other students.

Maiburg et al. (2003) designed a simulation of a general practitioner's consultation consisting of 12 interactive streaming-video patient cases presenting with complaints related to nutrition (i.e. food pyramid, obesity, diabetes mellitus, hypercholesterolemia, hypertension, irritable bowel syndrome, and constipation). After a plenary instruction session by the researcher, the GP trainees went through the program at their own pace during these sessions and this process took an average of 6 hours. The control group took the regular vocational training program but their knowledge did not increase as much as those using the program.

Whatever method students have used to learn, they need to revise before the summative assessment and it has been shown that nutrition students may benefit from the use of crossword puzzles that test their knowledge in an enjoyable way (Wise, 2001). The puzzles appear in a web page and students have to move the mouse over the first letter of a word to reveal the clue, some of which are cryptic and others simpler. They enter each letter by moving the mouse over the blank space on the screen and typing it. Students could not agree whether cryptic clues are enjoyable or whether puzzles are only worthwhile if clues are simple and not cryptic.

The strongest attitude shown by students was their strong agreement that crossword puzzles show them what they need to study more thoroughly. They also agreed that crossword puzzles: help with spelling of technical words, challenge students to answer without looking at their notes, help students to test their knowledge in a different format, give confidence that they have learned more than they realised when they can get the right answers, help them to concentrate on the material, give a sense of satisfaction when completed and help them to learn whilst having fun.

Computers are more often being used for distance learning and to replace lectures with self-study packages. Many different programs have been designed to provide formative feedback during learning. There are many different multiple-choice types of approach available and some of these may also be used for summative assessment at the end of courses. There are arguments against these simple programs though and it has been shown that through the use of feedback during study, students can improve weaknesses in learning and thinking, increase and transfer learning, and value opportunities to revise (Wang, 2007). Thus it is suggested that it is important for teachers to provide learners with opportunities for receiving 'timely feedback' and 'repeating the test'. When students have the opportunity to repeat the test, correct answers should not be given but only reference to where to find the answer. The program described automatically chooses some questions when the student logs in randomly from the database. A given test item will not show up on the following test if a learner correctly answers the test item three times consecutively.

Thus, the number of test items will gradually decrease with each iteration of the test. At some point, all questions will be answered correctly, and the system will tag the successful learner with a 'pass the test' mark. By the same token, if learners cannot answer the test item correctly three times consecutively, then the answer count will be reset to zero and begun again. Answering a test item correctly three times consecutively is considered necessary because the system judges that the learners may answer the question correctly simply by guessing. The purpose of this design is for learners to actively take on the challenge of learning, not passively guess their way through.

RESEARCH AND PLACEMENT

When students have undertaken sufficient education in nutrition, they may include in their course some experience of undertaking research and working in a placement. Student research projects can be enhanced by using a program that helps them write a protocol (Wise, 2002c). Important aspects of a research protocol include a definition of the research problem, sufficient detail about the plan of work, reasons for selecting the specified approach, and information related to how research funds will be allocated. The scientific method implies a logical derivation of conclusions by means of inference correctly drawn from reliable data. The analysis of experimental data is, therefore, a critical stage in every research study and statistical tests are required for most nutritional research and this should form an important part of the overall method described in the research protocol. At honours level, students have to design their own research project and write a simple research protocol to convince the supervisor that the student has sufficient understanding to design a study that is likely to be successful. It is useful practice for the possibility that the student will later be involved in actual research, to make this exercise as realistic as possible. In order to prompt the student to include the most important aspects of a research protocol, especially the statistical ones, a computer program has been developed. The student moves through various steps in which information is provided to remind the student about the relevant material taught earlier in the module on research methods. After filling in information and answering questions, the program writes a draft protocol suggesting a statistical test. The student is then expected to revise statistics sufficiently to be able to justify whether this is an appropriate test. The most positive feature of the program seen by the students was that it had 'links to useful material on the Internet'. There was also agreement that the program 'helps to clarify what is needed for my protocol', 'provoked me to think of aspects of the project, the importance of which I might have failed to realise early enough' and 'provoked me to ask appropriate questions of my supervisor about the project'.

Information technology can provide a learning experience whilst students are away from the university in a work placement. Kolasa et al. (2001) reported how medical students are expected to apply their nutritional knowledge by observing physicians on placement, but that students reported that few of their physician preceptors refer or counsel patients on dietary change. It was therefore decided to set up a discussion forum in which experienced physicians could reply to questions and points made by students whilst on placement. All questions were answered but many students apparently registered and only read the discussions without taking part themselves. Students were asked to evaluate the forum but only 10 of 72 medical students replied, but these were positive about the experience.

Another approach has been tried for our nutrition students in which they were encouraged to use a discussion forum to write about what they were doing on placement in a similar way to the report by McGugan & Peacock (2003). There were 9 nutrition students who undertook simultaneous placements in different work environments. Participation in the forum varied from only 2 communications from one student to 15 from the most prolific (see Figure 7). The most prolific student made the following comments on return from placement:

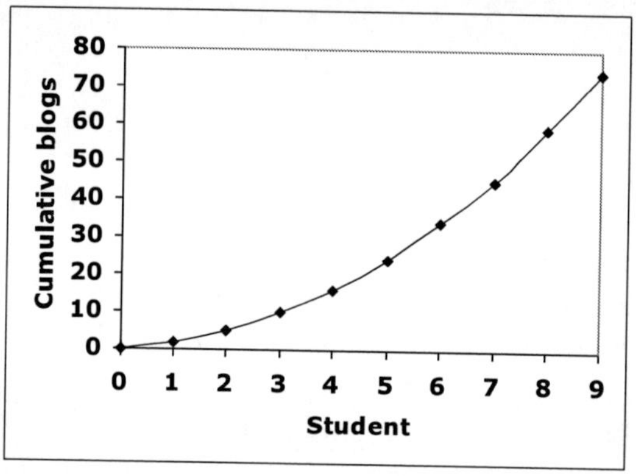

Figure 7. Cumulative graph to show contributions to a placement discussion forum by individual students

'I thought the discussion forum was a really good thing. It helped us stay in touch with each other over placement and learn about what else a nutritionist could be doing. I also think it helped me make a definite decision about the type of nutritionist career I wanted. The blogs I had written also helped with the placement report. While reading the blogs again, I remembered small bits and pieces that could go into the report.'

Conclusion

Information technology is useful for helping lecturers organise nutritional knowledge, animate presentations to make it clearer and interact with students. Various types of programs can be used to support self-study, for example of metabolism, research methods, dietary analysis, energy requirements for activity, and aspects of practice. The use of computers to enhance communication between students should also be considered, for example whilst they are on placement.

References

Department of Health (1991). Dietary Reference Values for Food Energy and Nutrients for the United Kingdom. London: HMSO.

eInstruction (2009). Interwrite responses assessment made simple. http://www.interwritelearning.com/products/response/benefits.html

Frey, B. A. & Birnbaum, D. J. (2002). Learners' perceptions on the value of PowerPoint in lectures. *Education Resources Information Center* ED467192.

Gachago, D. (2008). Feedback on Personal Response Systems ('Clickers') – lecturers' perspective. http://www.scieng.ed.ac.uk/LTStrategy/resources/Clicker_feedback_ v0_7_ incl _exec_summary.pdf

Garrow, J. S. (1978). Energy Balance and Obesity in Man. 2nd edn, pp. 119-121. Amsterdam: Elsevier/North-Holland Biomedical Press.

GenomeNet (2002). Kyoto encyclopedia of genes and genomes. http://www.genome.ad.jp/kegg/metabolism.html

Heath, D. (1995) An Introduction to Experimental Design and Statistics for Biology. London: UCL Press.

Herriot, A. M., Bishop, J. A. & Truby, H. (2004). The development and evaluation of Student Training, Education and Practice for Dietetics CD-ROM: a computer-assisted instruction programme for dietetic students. *Journal of Human Nutrition and Dietetics, 17*, 35–41.

Higher Education Academy (2009). Reward and recognition of teaching in higher education. http://www.heacademy.ac.uk/assets/York/documents/resources/publications/Reward_and_Recognition_Interim.pdf

Huck, S. W. & Cormier, W. H. (1996). Reading Statistics and Research. New York: Harper Collins Publishers Inc.

Kolasa, K. M., Daugherty, J. E., Jobe, A. C. & Miller, M. G. (2001). Virtual seminars for medical nutrition education: case example. *Journal of Nutrition Education, 33*, 347–351.

Kroeze. W., Werkma, A. & Brug, J. (2006). A systematic review of randomized trials on the effectiveness of computer-tailored education on physical activity and dietary behaviors. *Annals of Behavioural Medicine, 31*, 205-223.

Litchfield, R. E., Oakland, M. J. & Anderson, J. (2002). Promoting and evaluating competence in on-line dietetics education. *Journal of the American Dietetic Association, 102*, 1455-1458.

Maiburg, B. H. J., Rethans, J. J. E., Schuwirth, L. W. T., Mathus-Vliegen, L. M. H. & Van Ree, J. W. (2003). Controlled trial of effect of computer-based nutrition course on knowledge and practice of general practitioner trainees. *American Journal of Clinical Nutrition, 77*, 1019S–1024S.

McGugan, S. & Peacock, S. (2003). Research and evaluation into the role of computer-mediated conferencing and virtual learning environments to improve hospitality and tourism student supervision and peer support whilst on industrial placement. http://www.heacademy.ac.uk/assets/hlst/documents/projects/round_2/mcgugan_report.pdf

Nicholson, D. (2008) Making metabolism meaningful. *Centre for Bioscience Bulletin, 25*, 8.

Nutrition Society (2005). Professional nutrition education. http://www.nutritionsociety.org/documents/20060629nssubmissiontonutritio%20trainingreview.pdf

Roche Applied Science (2009). Biochemical pathways. http://www.expasy.ch/cgi-bin/search-biochem-index

Turner, R. E., Evers, W. D., Bennett Wood, O., Lehman, J. D. & Peck, L. W. (2000). Computer-based simulations enhance clinical experience of dietetics interns. *Journal of the American Dietetic Association, 100*, 183-190.

Wang, T. H. (2007). What strategies are effective for formative assessment in an e-learning environment? *Journal of Computer Assisted Learning, 23*, 171–186.

Wise, A. (2001). Web-based crossword puzzles support revision. *Active Learning in Higher Education, 2*, 180-188.

Wise, A. (2002a). Web-based program to illustrate metabolic pathways to students. CAL-laborate (June) 24-26.

Wise, A. (2002b). Web-based program to teach food composition. Proceedings of the Nutrition Society 61, 54A.

Wise, A. (2002c). A program to help students of life sciences prepare a research protocol. *Association of Learning Technology Journal, 10*, 83-89.

Wise, A. (2003) Web-based puzzle program to assist students' understanding of research methods. *Active Learning in Higher Education, 4*, 193-202.

Wise, A. (2006). Enhancement of a dietary analysis program to facilitate education. In Current Developments in Technology Assisted Education (2006) [A. Méndez-Vilas, A. Solano Martin, J. Mesa González and J.A. Mesa González, editors], pp. 816-820. Badajoz, Spain: Formatex.

Wise, A. (2008a). Transcriptional switches in the control of macronutrient metabolism. *Nutrition Reviews, 66*, 321–325.

Wise, A. (2008b). Developments in nutritional programming illustrated by WinDiets. *BNF Nutrition Bulletin, 33*, 55-57.

Wise, A. & Cowie, E. (2005). Activity diary program to enhance teaching of energy balance. Proceedings of the Science Learning and Teaching Conference 2005, 27-28 June 2005, University of Warwick, pp. 176-177.

In: Nutritional Education
Editor: Ida R. Laidyth

ISBN: 978-1-60876-078-7

Chapter 7

School Feeding Programmes for Improvement of School Children's Nutrition Status and School Attendance

Mary Walingo
School of Consumer Sciences & Tech, Maseno University, Maseno, Kenya

Abstract

School Feeding Programs have been established in most parts of the world with the goals of reducing hunger and malnutrition. School Feeding Programmes have potential to safeguard the health and the well-being of school children, and also promote good dietary, hygiene, and sanitation practices. School children grow up knowing the consumption of nutritious commodities and other foods. School Feeding Programs have been used as a means to distribute food to the pre-school and school-age children, as a food security net to improve their nutrition status, and also improve the general socio-economic conditions of rural communities as well as providing educational and nutritional benefits of participants. Nutrition status is a powerful determinant of educational health and developmental outcomes of school children. Nutrition status affects physical growth and maturation, and influences a person's attention span, learning capacity and ability to engage in educational experience. Undernutrition in early childhood has potential to negatively influence school aptitudes, time of school enrollment, school attendance and concentration. Schools provide an ideal channel for nutrition programs and services especially now that they reach many children. Acceptable dietary, hygiene and sanitation habits can be developed amongst school children in school. Most children from resource-poor households are often absent from schools as they provide child labor on farms and households to augment their families much needed income for food purchases. The development of health-promoting schools has promising returns for school children in developing countries. This study demonstrates the interaction of poverty, nutrition status and education. To improve the nutritional status and school attendance of the pupils whose parents cannot afford to participate in the School Lunch Programs, funding from external sources is essential. Efforts should be directed toward reducing hunger in the classroom and improving the nutritional status of pupils in schools. Inclusion of School Feeding Programs as a policy issue in national goals and objectives could result in improved nutritional status among school children.

INTRODUCTION

School Feeding Programs often occur through large organizations in collaboration with national governments and non-governmental organizations [Bennet, 2003; Tomlinson, 2007]. The UN World Food Program is the largest sponsor of these programs in many countries [United Nations/World Food Program (UN/WFP) 1992]. School Feeding Programs have been established in most parts of the world with the goals of reducing hunger and malnutrition. School Feeding Programmes have potential to safeguard the health and the well-being of school children, and also promote good dietary, hygiene, and sanitation practices, that result in a chain of Nutrition-Health schools for a healthy nation with developed capacity for work. School children grow up knowing the consumption of nutritious commodities and other foods. School Feeding Programs have been used as a means to distribute food to the pre-school and school-age children, as a food security net to improve their nutrition status [UN/WFP) 1992]. The School Lunch Program was enacted to enhance universal education for the socially disadvantaged and nutritionally vulnerable children, especially girls in primary and pre-primary schools in the Arid and Semi-Arid areas [Kuria, 2003].

The primary assumption of SFPs is based on the premise that learning and education depend on good nutrition. Further that good nutrition contributes to high enrolment rate, better school attendance and lower school drop-out rates, improved academic performance, social equity and general economic growth. Nutritional and health status are powerful influences on a child's learning and on how well a child performs in school. Sick and malnourished children do not have the same potential for learning as healthy normal children. Such children are usually from resource-poor households and suffer diminished cognitive development, and also reduced ability to participate in learning experiences.

The School Feeding Programs are designed to improve the general socio-economic conditions of rural communities as well as providing educational and nutritional benefits of participants [Dall Acqua, 1991]. Children from poor families are not only under-fed but also contribute to the household's economy, especially in terms of cheap labour, to supplement the meager and insufficient household incomes. These children are most likely to be absent from school, see no value for education and life..

School Feeding Programs in Kenya

School Feeding Programmes have been used as development intervention to improve the livelihoods of particular groups vulnerable to food insecurity [Bennet, 2003; Tomlinson, 2007]. These programmes were started as a joint venture in the Arid and semi-Arid lands and also in the less Arid and low potential areas by the Government of Kenya and the World Food Programme [United Nations/World Food Program (UN/WFP) 1992]. However the World Food Programme does not support the School Feeding Programmes in many parts of Kenya. In Kenya, School Feeding Programs in the Arid and Semi-Arid Areas and also in the less arid and low potential areas are sponsored by the Government of Kenya and the World Food Program (WFP) [Coursin, 1982]. In such programs the WFP seeks funding sources, provides food resources, repays 50% of transportation costs, and offers non-food resources.

The WFP does not support School Feeding Programs in Emuhaya District and other areas in Western Province of Kenya, Some Emuhaya District schools, through the Parent-Teacher Associations [PTA], organize School Lunch Programs that require parents or guardians of pupils to contribute either money or food (e.g. maize 4-6kgs and beans 6kgs) to support the Program. This arrangement is meant to save time for class and recreation during lunch hour, and to provide food to children whose mothers are not available to prepare lunch for their children. The meal is based on locally produced food and is intended to make up for possible food and nutrient imbalances in the children's daily diet. These programs seek to improve children's nutritional status, attendance levels, academic performance, school enrolment, and reduce the time spend by children going for lunch at home, and the distance travelled daily between home and school over lunch.

Western Province, especially Emuhaya District experiences food shortages almost throughout the year due to small farm sizes and high population density. School Lunch Programmes seek to reduce hunger among school children for effective learning [Coursin, 1982]. The meal provided should help school children to meet ⅓ to ¼ of their daily dietary requirements. Hunger in the classroom is generally believed to lead to lethargy, apathy and inability to pay attention [Coursin, 1982; Pollit, 1995]. These programmes are recognized as efficient networks to distribute food to the preschool and school age children [Tomlinson, 2007].

METHODS

The study was conducted in eight primary schools that had a School Lunch Program arrangement in Western Province of Kenya. Study subjects were classified into participants and non-participants of the School Lunch Program. The sample size was thus estimated at 320 pupils out of which 160 were participants and 160 were non-participants in the School Lunch Program. In each school a list of standard five and standard six pupils aged between 10 to 12 years was made and disaggregated between participants and non-participants in the School Lunch Program. A total of 40 pupils were selected from each of the eight study schools, making a total sample of 320 pupils.

Qualification for inclusion in the study as a SLP participant was based on a pupil's participation in the School Lunch Program for at least two continuous years to enable assessment of the dietary effects on nutritional status. The measure of the program participation was consumption of the school lunch for five consecutive days in a school week, and was based on usual School Lunch Program participation practices. Interviews were arranged with each respondent on scheduled days. The researchers went to each pupil's home to collect data from the pupils and their caregivers. Caregivers were interviewed regarding their socio-economic status, their child's school attendance, their opinion about the school lunch, and food frequency intake. School registers provided by the class teacher were also used to extract information about the students' school attendance record.

A twenty-four hour diet recall was used to gather dietary intake data for home food intake of participants and nonparticipants. The twenty-four hour diet recall survey was used to establish the meal patterns, estimate the level of energy and protein intake of pupils, and establish the adequacy of home meals. The contribution of the School Lunch to the participants' daily nutrient intake was assessed by weighing the volume of food portions served, consumed and leftover by each participating student. The proportions of ingredients used in cooking the School Lunch and the total volume cooked were also recorded. The food consumption data from the 24-hour recall and School Lunch of each pupil was converted manually into energy and protein intakes using the food composition tables for Kenya [Sehmi, 1993]. Dietary adequacy of the participants and nonparticipants was assessed by comparison of their protein and energy intake with the Dietary Reference Intakes [National Academy of Sciences, 2008].

The pupil's nutrition status was assessed by comparing the pupil's age, weight and height measurements computed as weight-for-age, height-for-age and weight-for-height with the reference values of the United States National Centre for Health Statistics (NCHS) using the Epi-Info program [Version 6.0, Centers for Disease Control, Atlanta, GA, USA]. Underweight [low weight-for-age], stunting [low height-for-age] and wasting [low weight-for-height] were defined as proportions of pupils who had index scores falling below -2SD of the NCHS mean.

Data were entered and analyzed by the Statistical Package for Social Sciences [SPSS] program [Windows version 9.0, Chicago, IL, USA]. Percentages and means [and standard deviations] were computed for continuous variables, while frequencies were computed for categorical variables. Associations between nutrition indices and school lunch variables were tested by Chi Square (χ^2) while the Independent-samples t-test was used to compare group means for significance.

RESULTS AND DISCUSSION

Socioeconomic Characteristics of Households of Pupils

Socioeconomic characteristics of the caregivers of pupils attending schools were categorized into marital status, level of education and occupation of the head of household, and the average household monthly income. While fewer (6.3%0 and separated (5%) of pupils were single (13.1%) and 18.1% were separated. Further 11.3% of families with non-participating pupils were divorced. It seems participation of pupils in the school lunch is affected by the stability of their families in terms of marital status. Settled or married families tend to (χ^2 =25.39, DF=1) make decisions that favour participation of pupils in the school programs. Caregivers whose pupils did not participate in the SLP were less likely to be married, had a lower education level and lower income.

More parents of participating pupils had attained better levels of education than those of non-participating pupils (χ^2 =14.02, DF=1) Among the families with participant pupils 9.4% had no formal education and 20% had primary education, while among the non-participant group 18.1% had no formal education and 31% had primary education. More children from the non-participant group came from families where parents were either teachers (29.4%0 compared 18.8%), or were in small trade (35.6%) compared to 32.5% families from the participant group. While 29.9% families of non-participant pupils were farmers and 8.1% involved in other activities, 29.4% families of participant pupils were farmers and 19.4% were involved in other economic activities. About 23.8% families of participant pupils had a total monthly income of Kshs 5000, 32.5% had income ranging between 5001-7500 and 43.7% had Kshs 7500. About 44.4% families of non-participant pupils had a total monthly income of Kshs 5000, 26.9% had income ranging between 5001-7500 and 28.8% had Kshs 7500. Families of participant pupils had higher income compare to those of non-participant pupils (χ^2 =16.85 DF=1)

The income level, level of education and nature of occupation of the caregivers influenced pupils' participation in the School Lunch Program. The unemployed caregivers had difficulties in meeting the participation criteria. The level of education of the caregivers of participant pupils, though low, was better than that of caregivers of nonparticipant pupils. The low literacy levels observed in the population could reduce the caregivers' understanding of the role of School Lunch in the physical and mental development of a child. The educated caregivers are likely to be more knowledgeable about nutrition requirements of children which may result in better childhood feeding practices. The level of education of caregivers is also likely to determine their occupation and influence income level.

Pupil participation in the SLP is influenced by the ability of families to meet the participation criteria which requires families to pay a fee for the School Lunch and contribute maize and beans. Nonparticipant families who find great difficulties in meeting their basic needs including education of their children may remain poor through many generations if adequate targeted interventions are not addressed. Intervention efforts directed at strengthening the School Lunch Programs, to include more children from poor families, and also increase variety of the School Lunch could have promising returns by improving both the nutritional status and school attendance of pupils. Funding for School Feeding Programmes can relieve some of the families' burden of sharing their scarce financial resources between competing basic household demands and thereby improve the nutrition status of their children.

Parents Opinion about the School Lunch

Open-ended questions were given to assess the caregivers' opinion about the School Lunch. About 46% of the caregivers (n=147) indicated that the conditions for participation in the School Lunch Program were not favorable for their economic status. Thirty-two percent of non-participating caregivers indicated that their children could go home to eat lunch but 12% did not think lunch was an important meal. Among the parents who reported that the school lunch was too expensive, 22% of them reported that their children could carry snacks to school. Almost half of the non-participating caregivers (44%) thought that the School Lunch improved children's nutritional status and 17% indicated that it encouraged regular school attendance by their children. Thirteen percent of caregivers stated that the school lunch saved their children from walking long distances to their homes to eat lunch, and these parents indicated that the long distances children walked back home for lunch could cause fatigue and reduce their concentration levels during lessons.

Effect of the School Lunch on Attendance and Enrollment

Class registers were examined to assess levels of school attendance of participant and nonparticipant pupils, as measured by the number of times a student stayed away from school. Participant pupils attended school more regularly than the nonparticipant pupils (χ^2= 29.98, DF=1). The nonparticipant pupils missed school because of sickness (18.7%), lack of school requirements (20%), hunger (53.8%), and other reasons such as helping caregivers in domestic chores and taking care of their younger siblings (7.5%). The participant pupils missed school due to sickness (72.2%), hunger (2.8%), and other reasons such as helping caregivers in domestic chores and taking care of their younger siblings (25%). Hunger was a significant reason for missing school among the nonparticipant pupils (χ^2 = 69.13, DF=4). The level of school attendance was higher among pupil participants than the non-participant pupils. Hungry children suffer less concentration and have difficulties performing complex tasks. Temporary hunger is common in children who are not fed before going to school and has adverse effect on learning. There is improved performance on short-term memory test and discrimination of geometric patterns, especially among malnourished children under breakfast conditions [Pollit, 1995].

About 13% of the nonparticipant pupils walked long distances to eat the home lunch while those nonparticipants who cannot reach their homes remained hungry and yet were expected to attend the afternoon classes. Many factors contribute to hunger among school children. For example children travel long distances to school, the food habits of a people that include no or small breakfast, lack of family time or resources to provide adequate meals to children.

School Feeding Programs increase enrolment and attendance in schools, particularly amongst girls [Bennett, 2003; Bundy, 2005; Miller Del Rosso, 1999; Tomlison, 2007]. Food can act as an incentive for children to attend school regularly, with girls receiving the most benefits as parents see sufficient income-transfer benefits from the school meal. School Lunch Programs have been reported to stabilize attendance and increase enrollment in Kenya [de Moel *et al*, 1997] and India [Babu and Hallam, 1989].

Investment School Feeding Programs contribute to cognitive attentiveness, improved school attendance, and reduced absenteeism and better household food security. Among well-nourished children a nineteen to twenty hour fasting period affects attention, and the capacity to solve problems of visual perceptual organization. Increasing attention may have significant education benefits in the long run by ensuring that the exposure of the student to the materials taught in schools. The SFPs alleviate short-term hunger [Pollit, 1995], that could affect the learning capacity of children.

Weekly Food Frequency Consumption of Participant and Nonparticipant Pupils

The weekly food frequency consumption survey did not demonstrate significant differences between food consumption patterns of families of participating and nonparticipating students with the exception that vegetable consumption was greater in families with participants. Three meals were served each day; breakfast, lunch and supper.

Foods commonly served for breakfast included porridge, or tea, served with either bread, boiled or fried bananas, boiled cassava, or boiled sweet potatoes. Only 17 % of all the pupils did not take breakfast. The home lunch was composed of porridge and tea, served with either boiled/fried bananas, boiled cassava, arrowroots or boiled sweet potatoes. About 72% of the nonparticipant pupils walked back home to eat lunch while 12% did not eat lunch. While 24% ate rice with bean stew, only 14% ate the staple food, *ugali,* served with either a vegetable relish or beef stew.

Caregivers contributed to the school lunch by providing an agreed upon amount of maize (4 kgs) and beans (4 kgs) per child per school term, usually 12 weeks of continuous learning. The school diet consisted of boiled maize and beans fried in vegetable oil. Each school pooled together the contributions of the caregivers to the school lunch.

Foods consumed by school children ranged from boiled maize and beans, ugali, boiled sweet potatoes, boiled cassava, boiled or fried green bananas, bean stew, green gram stew and arrowroots. These foods were generally rich in carbohydrates with a high satiety value and were affordable unlike foods rich in proteins which were expensive. Intake of cereals, and, roots and tubers was higher in the non-participants than in the participants, while the intake of legumes, vegetables, fruits, meats, and fats and oils was higher in the participants. Except for the intake of vegetables which was significantly higher in the participating group, the intake of other foods was not significantly different among the two groups. Fruits were consumed only in a small number of the households and the level of consumption is still below the DRI (table 1).

Vegetables and fruits known to be rich in vitamins, minerals and phytochemicals of health value were not served in most household diets and in the school lunch, and thus a dietary deficiency in most minerals and vitamins.

The commonly consumed vegetables included kales and a range of indigenous vegetables. Vegetables and fruits are a good source of micronutrients and phytochemicals of good health and nutritional value, and confer protection against infections by boosting the immune system. The food diversity index was low indicating lack of variety in the foods consumed by children from both groups. Children ate monotonous diets that were low in energy and protein, and could predispose them to micronutrient deficiencies.

Table 1. Weekly food consumption frequency for pupils in households

Foods	Participants (No. of times/week)	Non-Participants (No. of times/week)	P-Value
Cereals	17.4	18.4	NS
Legumes/pulses	16.0	15.2	NS
Milk and milk products	7.8	6.8	NS
Fats and Oils	4.1	4.0	NS
Vegetables	5.2*	2.8	3.8*
Meats	1.8	1.5	NS
Fruits	0.7	0.0	NS
Roots and tubers	7.2	7.9	NS

Note: * - Significant P<0.05

NS – Not significant

Agriculture biodiversity of a household has an influence on the diversity of diets given to children [Rainville, 2001]. The diversity of meals given to preschool children is low and diets lack variety of foods. Children consume inadequate and monotonous diets that are mainly composed of carbohydrates and are low in micronutrients. Such diets predispose children to several aspects of immunocompetence such as cell-mediated immunity, osponization and mucosal immunity [Gordon, Devaney and Burghardt, 1995]. The objective of the study was to assess the effect of a School Lunch Feeding Program on food and nutrient intake of school age children participating in the program.

The average energy and protein quantity of the school lunch was 841 Kcal and 40g protein per student per day. Increasing variety of foods across and within groups is important for adequate nutrition. Lunch and super contributed higher amounts of nutrients (24% of energy and 17.7% of the total protein for participants and 20.4% energy and 17.7% for non-participants) to the total daily nutrient intake in both groups. The lunch energy intake (841±107.5) of participants was higher (T-value 63.24) than that of the non-participants (720±140), and protein intake (40±3.24) of participants was higher (T-value 15.84) than that of the non-participants (24±44.1). These intakes contributed to more than 30% of the DRI for both energy and protein.

The contribution to Dietary Reference Intake for energy was (35.04±4.48%) for participants and (30.0±5.83%) and for protein was (117.6±9.52%) for the participants and (70.6±129.71%) for the non-participants. Dietary Reference Intake for energy 2089±310.25 for participants and 1841±392, and the intake were higher among the participants (T-value 87.67). The DRI for protein intake was 170.6±9.94 for the participants and 117.6±3.18 for the non-participants and was significantly higher among the participants (T-value 15.68). The School Lunch made a significant contribution to the nutrient intake of the pupils. Energy and protein consumption of pupil participants was higher than that of the pupil nonparticipants and the nonparticipants were more likely to report being hungry.

The difference in energy and protein intake at lunch between participating and non-participating children could be attributed to the School Lunch Programme providing higher amount of the nutrients than the Home Lunch. However, though the school lunch contributed significantly to the total daily nutrient intake of participants, their caloric intake was still low. The school lunch played a significant role in contributing more than $^{1}/_{3}$ of RDA for nutrients and to the overall diet adequacy of the participants. Foods provided for school age children should satisfy the high demands of rapid growth, intense physical activity and mental development, besides guarding against diseases.

Studies on impact of School Lunch Programs on students' dietary intakes have reported increased intakes of energy [Mathews, 1996; Gleason and Suitor, 2008] and protein [Mathews, 1996; Gleason and Suitor, 2008; Ho *et al*, 1991; Gleason and Suitor, 2003; Rainville, 2001].]. Some researchers [Ho *et al*, 1991; Rainville, 2001] have reported less consumption of energy among participant students' in the School Lunch programs. In Peru, children who received breakfast at schools in the treatment group had increased dietary intakes of energy, protein and iron [Jacobey and Cueto and Pollit, 1996]. Children with low calorie intake over long periods of time reach a state of energy balance through reductions in activity level, and thus a loss of significant opportunities for learning.

Nutrition Status of Pupils

Nutritional status indicators of School Lunch participants were categorized into underweight, stunting and wasting. Severe underweight, severe stunting and severe wasting were significantly higher among the nonparticipants than among the participants. Parents' income had a significant relationship to the nutritional status of pupils, but the amount of land owned and food crop production levels in families did not have a significant influence on the nutritional status of pupils. The level of education and nature of occupation of the parent were positively associated with weight-for-age and height-for-age of the participant pupils. Pupils from households where parents were in wage employment (42.6%) tended to be of a significantly better nutritional status than those whose parents were not employed. The nutritional status of pupils who participated in the School Lunch Program was better than that of nonparticipating students. Severe underweight, severe stunting and severe wasting were significantly higher among the pupil nonparticipants.

A hungry child has decreased ability to learn and also suffer reduced concentration in class. Providing breakfast to primary school students significantly increased attendance and arithmetic scores, and mostly benefited children who were stunted, wasted or previously malnourished [Cullen, Watson and Zakeri, 2007]. Breakfast programs are beneficial to nutrient intake, school attendance and academic performance Pollit, 1995].

School Lunch Programs reportedly increase intakes of energy and protein [Babu Hallam, 1989; Cullen, Watson, and Zakeri, 2007; Pollit, 1995; Mathews 1996; Gleason and Suitor 2001; Ho, Gould and Jensen *et al,* 1991] in other parts of the world. Results of an assessment of the quality of a School Lunch Programme in New York among 1600 black children revealed gain in stature and weight among school children who ate the school lunch than those who ate either at home or at nearby shops [Gleason and Suitor, 2003].

Nutrition status is a powerful determinant of educational health and developmental outcomes of school children. Nutrition status affects physical growth and maturation, and influences a person's attention span, learning capacity and ability to engage in educational experience [Pollit, 1990: Levinger 1996, and WHO 1996].

Conclusion, Recommendation and Emerging Issues

The School Lunch Programme provided more energy and protein to participants than the lunch given to non-participants at home. There was more variety in the foods consumed by the participants than the non-participants, although they both had a low variety index. There is a synergistic interaction between poverty, nutrition status and school attendance that finally impact the whole education system. Poor nutrition among school children is a causal factor to inefficiency and non-performance in the education sector in developing communities.

Undernutrition in early childhood has potential to negatively influence school aptitudes, time of school enrollment, school attendance and concentration. Pupils of a poor nutrition status are more likely to suffer high morbidity rates that keep them out of school contributing to absenteeism and discontinued learning. These children are also at increased risk of high drop-out rates, and start school when they are much older compared to the normal children. The future national human resource capital formation is thoroughly compromised due to the diminished work capacity of its population and increased expenditure o limited national resources on health.

The irregular school of malnourished and unhealthy children is one of the key factors in poor performance. To improve the nutritional status and school attendance of the pupils whose parents cannot afford to participate in the School Lunch Programs, funding from external sources is essential. Efforts should be directed toward reducing hunger in the classroom and improving the nutritional status of pupils in schools. Inclusion of School Feeding Programs as a policy issue in national goals and objectives could result in improved nutritional status among school children.

There is need for the Government intervention to subsidize meals to schools to widen participation to include much poorer pupils whose energy intake is below the RDA. The school Lunch Programmes should be used as networks for food distribution to children as a form of family relief to poor parents to enable them reallocate their meagre resources to other competing household demands. There is need to vary the meals served to children to include a variety of cereals, legumes, fruits and vegetables which can be grown in the School garden. Establishment of school gardens can be an important source of food to combat some of the nutrition-related diseases.

Understanding the nutrient adequacy of meals consumed by school children is necessary to inform on the role of diet in the development of diet-related diseases in the population.

Schools provide an ideal channel for nutrition programs and services especially now that they reach many children. Acceptable dietary, hygiene and sanitation habits can be developed amongst school children in school. Most children from resource-poor households often are absent from schools as they provide child labor on farms and households to enhance their households much needed income for food purchases.

The development of nutrition and health-promoting schools has promising returns for school children in developing countries. Model projects can be tested to ascertain the advantage of health-promoting school's policies and practices in line with the existing national policies.

References

[1] Babu, SC; Hallam JA. Socioeconomic impacts of School Feeding Programs: Empirical evidence from a south Indian village. *Food Policy*. 1989, 14, 58-66.

[2] Bennett, J. Review of School Feeding Projects. Department for International Development. September 2003

[3] Bundy, D. School Health and Nutrition: Policy and Programs. *Food and Nutrition Bulletin*, Vol 26, no 2(supplement 2) 2005, The United Nations University.

[4] Coursin, D. Report on Nutrition, Brain Development and Behavior. New York: MacMillan Co. 1982.

[5] Cullen, K; Watson, K; Zakeri, I. Impact of National School Lunch Program Meal and Competitive foods. Middle school Student Lunch Consumption. United States Department of Agriculture, Food Assistance and Nutrition Research Program. Economic Research Service 2007.

[6] Dall Acqua, FM. Economic adjustment and nutrition policies: Evaluation of a school-lunch program in Brazil. *Food Nutr Bull.* 1991, 13, 202-209.

[7] De Moel, JPC; Pietters, JJL; Van Der Hoeven, WJM. Effects of school feeding on growth of children in Kirinyaga District, Kenya. *E Afr Med J.* 1997, 54, 624-629.

[8] Gleason, P; & Suitor, C. Children's Diets in the Mid-1990's: Dietary intake and its relationship with school meal participation. Report No. CN-01-CD1, USDA, Food and Nutrition Service. 2001. www.ers.usda.gov/publications/ccr30/ccr30.pdf. Accessed February 15, 2008.

[9] Gleason, P; & Suitor, C. Eating at school: How the National School Lunch Program affects children's diets. *Am. J. Agric. Econ.*, 2003, 85, 1047-1061.

[10] Gordon, AR; Devaney, BI; Burghardt, JA. Dietary effects of the National School Lunch Program and the School Breakfast Program. *Am J Clin Nutr.*, 1995, 61, 205S–212S.

[11] Ho, CS; Gould, RA; Jensen, LN., *et al,* Evaluation of the nutrient content of school snack and vending lunch of junior high school students. *School Food Service Review..* 1991, 15 (2), 85-90.

[12] Jacobey, E; Cueto, S; Pollit, E. Benefits of a School Breakfast Program among Andean children in Huaraz, Peru. *Food and Nutrition Bulletin.* 1996, 17, 54-61.

[13] Kuria, EN. School Nutrition Programs in Kenya: Challenges and Opportunities. A paper presented to: Global Child Nutrition Forum and ASFSA: *Annual National Conference, Reno Nevada.,* USA on 17th – 23rd July 2003.

[14] Mathews, R. Importance to breakfast to cognitive performance and health. *Perspectives in Applied Nutrition.* 1996, 33, 204-212.

[15] Miller Del Rosso, J. 1999, June. School Feeding Programs: Improving Effectiveness and Increasing the Benefit to Education. A guide for Program Managers.

[16] National Academy of Sciences. Institute of Medicine. Dietary Reference Intakes: Recommended Intakes for Individuals. Available at: http://www.iom.edu/Object.File/Master/21/372/0.pdf. Accessed March 7, 2008.

[17] Pollit, E. Does breakfast make a difference in school? *J Am Diet Assoc.*, 1995, 95, 1134-1139.

[18] Rainville, AJ. Nutritional quality of reimbursable School Lunches compared to lunches brought from home in elementary schools in two South Eastern Michigan Districts. *J Child Nutr Man.* 2001, 25, 13-18.

[19] Sehmi, KJ. National food composition tables and the planning of satisfactory diets in Kenya. 1993. Government Printers, Nairobi, Kenya.

[20] Tomlinson, M. School Feeding in East and Southern Africa: Improving food sovereignty or photo opportunity? Regional Network for Equity in Southern Africa [EQUINET] EQUINET Discussion Paper No. 46. 2007 Health Systems Research Unit, Medical Research council.

[21] United Nations/World Food Program (UN/WFP), Food Assistance to Pre-Primary and Primary Schools. Ministry of Planning and National Development. 1992 Nairobi, Kenya.

[22] WHO East, Central and Southern Africa Food Composition Tables. Geneva: WHO 1997.

In: Nutritional Education
Editor: Ida R. Laidyth

ISBN: 978-1-60876-078-7

Chapter 8

MATERNAL NUTRITIONAL EDUCATION BEFORE AND DURING PREGNANCY

Hiroko Watanabe*

School of Medicine Faculty of Nursing, Shiga Medical Science
Seta Tsukinowa-cho, Otsu, Shiga, 520-2192 Japan

ABSTRACT

Maternal nutritional status before and during pregnancy constitutes one of the most important determinants for fetal growth. In adequate body weight before conception and low maternal weight gain are associated with adverse perinatal outcomes. The fetal origins hypothesis proposes that inadequate maternal nutrition and a low infant birth weight can predispose the child to diseases such as, diabetes and cardiovascular disease later in life. Pregnancy can be an opportune time to improve nutrition, and presents an ideal time for health promotion activities. However, many women of childbearing age do not maintain good nutritional status before and during pregnancy. They do not have an opportunity to get adequate and appropriate nutrition education in antenatal care. Most of them expect advice on general dietary improvements, with the remainder seeking advice on helping to promote their quality and quantity of nutritional intake. All women of reproductive age should be encouraged to follow the Government recommendation and eat a well-balanced diet. Health care providers need to ensure pregnant women know the positive and negative effect of poor maternal nutrition status, including the need for additional folate, at each physical check-up. An individualized approach is likely to have better outcomes than a standard intervention that is given to all pregnant women. A critical goal to achieve is for women to make behavior changes for good nutritional status before, during, and beyond pregnancy, which may lead to improved birth outcomes.

* Corresponding author: Tel: +81-77-548-2433. Fax: +81-77-548-2433, E-mail: watana@belle.shiga-med.ac.jp

COMMENTARY

Evidence indicates that women with a normal prepregnancy body mass index (BMI) and those who meet the recommended weight gains are healthiest and have healthier children. Maternal nutrition may be a key factor influencing the health of women during pregnancy and the development of the fetus. Therefore, health care providers expect that pregnancy can be an opportune time to improve nutrition, and presents an ideal time for health promotion activities. In addition, they expect that not only pregnant women to be concerned about their nutrition for giving birth to healthy newborns, but also that young women who expect to be mothers in the future will try to eat a well balanced diet. Promoting good health and nutrition before conception may be at least as important as during pregnancy. However, the condition of women must be changed including body composition, eating habits, and management of weight gain.

Changes in Body Composition for Women of Reproductive Age

Maternal size before conception plays a key role in determining the perinatal outcomes. High prepregnancy BMI, overweight and obesity, is a risk factor for adverse pregnancy outcomes, such as gestational diabetes, preeclampsia, cesarean delivery, and having a macrosomic [Kabiru and Raynor, 2004]. An increase of prepregnancy BMI was reported in the USA, and about one-third of all pregnant women are obese. Fifty % of African American women, 40% of Hispanic women, and 30% of white women are obese. In addition, one-third of adolescents are classified as either overweight or obese [Ogden et al., 2008].

Overall, the prevalence of prepregnancy overweight has increased steadily among low income black, Hispanic, and white women in the United States. Similar trends have been observed in Europe, e.g., in Sweden and Switzerland [Berg et al., 2005]. Between 1992 and 2002, the incidence of overweight in women of childbearing age increased from 6.8% to 19.3% for women aged 14-24 years, from 11.8% to 19.3% for those aged 25-34, and from 18.0% to 24.8% for those aged 35-44. In the UK, 33% of women are overweight and 23% obese [RCOG, 2006]. The burden of nutritional problems may be shifting from energy imbalance deficiency to excess among adolescents in these developed countries. Weight gain has been attributed more to decreasing levels of physical activity than to increased energy intake. Thus, perhaps lowered energy expenditure is the major factor in the higher levels of obesity.

On the other hand, industrialized countries face not only the epidemic of obesity, but also face underweight in women of reproductive age. Low prepregnancy BMI has been associated with a higher incidence of miscarriage [Helgstrand and Anderson, 2005], the delivery of smaller infants [Sekiya et al., 2007], and intrauterine growth restriction [Eherenberg et al., 2003].The highest prevalence of underweight was observed in younger women and Asian women. The prevalence of underweight women has increased 19.6% to 21.2% in the age of 20-29 years, and 8.6% to 13.3% in the ages of 30-39 during the last two decades in Japan. A low body mass index in highly industrialized countries cannot be considered to be a result of environmental factors such as periodic food shortages and malnutrition, but as an expression of constitutional low weight or a result of cosmetically-induced starvation. Bringing maternal weight into a health range before pregnancy makes conception easier, improving pregnancy outcomes.

Current Maternal Nutritional Status

Maternal nutritional status before and during pregnancy constitutes one of the most important determinants for fetal growth. Lower intake of calories, grams of food, protein, and carbohydrates are associated with inadequate pregnancy weight gain [NRCIM, 2007]. On the other hand, high intake of calories leading to excessive weight gain has been associated with long-term obesity risks, and postpartum retention [Polley et al., 2002]. A good diet should provide the amount and variety of nutrients to ensure optimal health for both mother and baby. Each country issues recommended dietary allowance (RDA) as the mean of estimated requirements for pregnant women, which needs to be increased to meet the demands of increasing maternal tissues, growth of the fetus, growing fat stores and the increase in basal metabolic rate (Table 1). .

Table1. Nutrient demands of pregnant women according to WHO, EU, USA and Japan

	Additional energy. kcal/d	Proteins g/d	Calcium mg/d	Iron mg/d	Folic acid μ g/d
WHO		51	1,000-1,200	12.5	370-470
Europe	200‡	48-60	700	17-21	400
USA	340†, 452‡	71	1,000	27-30	600
Canada	300† ‡		1,000	27	600
India		65	1,000	38	400
Japan	350†, 500‡	60	600-700	19.5	440

† : in the second trimester

‡ : in the third trimester

Nutrient intake data from studies of pregnant women are summarized in Table 2. The mean energy intake was greater than the RDA in some studies, but not other micronutrient intakes. This over-nutrition and imbalanced diet can contribute, potentially to excessive gestational weight gain. On the other hand, consistent with the report of the American Dietetic Association that many women of childbearing age do not maintain good nutritional status during pregnancy [Kaiser et al., 2008], mean energy intake tended to be lower than the RDA in some studies, especially among women with low income, having a low birth weight, living in a rural area, or being at a younger age. Furthermore, the mean intake of calcium and iron was observed less than the RDA or close to the RDA.

One of the important micronutrients is folate, which can reduce the risk of neural tube defects (NTD), low birth weight of infants, and recurrent spontaneous abortion. A significant low mean folic acid intake was observed among younger women, multiparous, and poorly educated women from low income families [Gautam et al., 2008]. However, mean dietary

Table 2. Reported average nutrient intakes during pregnancy in industrialized and developing countries

Country and Reference	Number of subjects	Energy kcal/d	Proteins g/d	Calcium mg/d	Iron mg/d	Folic acid µg/d	Dietary assessment
USA Fowles ER et al. 2009	n=13, 19-31 years old, first trimester	2653		961	20	387	24h dietary recall
USA Rifas-Shiman SL et al. 2006	n=1543, 16-45 years old, second trimester	2137±640		1168±344	16.7±5.9	367±134	semi-quantative FFQ
USA Siega-Riz AM et al. 2002	n=1131Non-Hispanic white women	2530±1192	94±42.1		18.2±8.8	604±284	FFQ
	n=971 Non-Hispanic black women, second trimester	3220±172	115±64.1		22.3±12.5	736±432	
Canada Pick ME et al. 2005	n=52, 21-41 years old, second or third trimester	2309±53.4		1,139±46.6	15.9±0.6	331±12.2	4-day food records
UK Rees GA et al. 2005	165 women with LBW infants n=63 Caucasian	1832	68.0	780	10.7	227	food records
	n=36 African	1586	62.1	565	9.6	196	
	n=26 Asian	1750	67.5	629	11.7	217	
	n=40 African-Caribbean	1740	65.4	658	9.8	189	
UK Ford et al. 2008	n=83, low income women 22±5 years old	1864.2± 501.9[a]	59±17	720±276		217±76	FFQ
UK Mouratidou et al. 2006	n=250, 14-18 weeks, 15-43 years old	1880	74.2	692	10.2	204	FFQ
Germany Franke et al. 2008	Mean age 30.8 years old, third trimester n=68 Germany	2203				254	FFQ
	n=147 Spain	2934				304	
	n= 55 Hungary	2926				396	
Greek Petrakos et al. 2006	n=98, second trimester			1216±555.9	11.6±5.0	341.5± 119.1	semi-quantative questionnaire
	n=102, third trimester			1282.5± 546.3	11.9±4.9	351.1± 155.0	
Kenya Kamau-Mbuthia et al. 2007	n=716	2055±537	59.3± 22.4	441±386	16.1±5.4		24-hour food recall
India Agrahar-Murugkar et al. 2004	19-40 years old, second or third trimester n=52 low-income pregnant	2418.7± 121.9	60.2± 4.7	434.9± 111.0	17.4±2.6		FFQ
	n=26 high-income pregnant	2633.8± 328.1	77.0± 14.9	456.1± 145.7	23.2±7.5		
India Gautam VP et al. 2008	n=114, living in rural villages 12 to 20th weeks	1541± 410.1	47.1± 13.9		15.0±6.4	152.2± 72.4	FFQ

Table 2. (Continued)

Country and Reference	Number of subjects	Energy kcal/d	Proteins g/d	Calcium mg/d	Iron mg/d	Folic acid µg/d	Dietary assessment
Japan Takimoto et al, 2003	n=330, 20-49 years old	1869±498	73.7± 22.8	597.7± 296.8	11.0±4.6		food weighing
Japan Watanabe et al. 2008	n=197, 19-42 years old, second trimester	1754.8± 442.3	57.1± 21.5	521.5± 213.4	6.1± 1.9	261.6± 94.3	FFQ

Values are presented as mean±SD
FFQ: food frequency questionnaire
a:7.8MJ

folate intake is barely half of the recommended values and at an extremely lowlevel in almost all studies during the 2000's.

A variety of methods have been developed for use in the assessment of nutrient status. As see in the Table 2, nutritional status was evaluated by a food frequency questionnaire (FFQ) on food recall or food weighing in the studies. Weighed food records, which are considered to be the gold standard of dietary assessment methodologies and provide a more precise estimation of an individual's actual nutrient intake, are associated with a large respondent burden, low response rate, and possible impact on usual food consumption. The FFQ gives useful estimates of nutrient intakes in pregnant women and the FFQ is a valid tool compared with 24 recalls. Nevertheless, over-reporting of nutritional habits and an underestimation of undesirable habits cannot be completely ruled out. The reliability of the self reported data depends on whether participants are able to accurately recall past behaviors. In addition, the data in Table 2 is not broadly representative of most women of reproductive age in each country due to the limited sample number, and the lack of information about physical activity. Therefore, we should carefully evaluate the observed nutritional intake values.

Assessment of nutritional status is only evaluated by gestational and weekly weight gain, and nutritional intake. However, we should be more concerned about biochemical assessments for poor control of weight gain or poor nutritional status, such as plasma ketone levels, which are elevated with poor nutrition or poor diabetic control. Hyperketonemia can progress to the accelerated starvation of pregnancy should caloric intake be deficient [Knopp, 1997]. Plasma ketone levels may useful as indicators of inappropriate weight control for diabetic women, but also for all pregnant women for weight control.

Optimal Weight Gain Management

Adequate weight gain is important for optimal perinatal outcomes. Some countries have devised pregnancy weight gain guidelines by prepregnancy BMI. Weight gain within the guidelines has been associated with healthy fetal and maternal outcomes. Weight gain below the goals is associated with low neonatal birth weight, and weight gain above the goals is associated with neonatal macrosomia [Parker and Abrams, 1992]. Not only is excessive weight gain responsible for complications during pregnancy, it also contributes to increased postpartum weight retention.

The 1990 Institute of Medicine (IOM) recommendations, shown in Table 3, have been the standard for weight gain during pregnancy since 1990 [IOM, 1990]. Shieve et al. [1998]

reported that two thirds of women gain more weight in pregnancy than is recommended by the IOM. Stotland et al. [2006] examined in 20,463 women with term singleton births, and reported that 43% of women gained weight above the recommended IOM range, whereas 37% gained within the IOM range, and 20% had weight gains below the target range. In a study of over 4000 women from the University of California, San Francisco Perinatal Database, 23% of underweight women, 49% of normal-weight women, and 70% of overweight women exceeded the recommendations [Carmichael et al., 1997]. These results suggest that the intervention including nutritional education, behavioral strategies to promote healthy and appropriate weight gain during pregnancy, was not effective for the targeted groups.

The recommendation may be not applicable to all women of reproductive age. Maternal anthropometry differs across race and age. The number of adolescent, Asian, Hispanics, and black women is increased. The recommendation must be set up for understanding their characteristics and a different classification of prepregnancy BMI needs to be applied. The current recommendations need to be updated, specifically for obese women and adolescents, because the 1990 recommendations did not consider the effect of weight gain on maternal outcomes of pregnancy. A produce ethnic-specific maternal weight gain recommendations is needed.

Table 3. Recommended gestational weight gains based on prepregnancy BMI

Prepregnancy BMI	BMI category	Recommended total weight gain	
		(kg)	(lb)
Less 19.8	Under weight	12.5-18	28-40
19.8 to 26.0	Normal	11.5-16	25-35
26.1 to 29.0	Overweight	7-11.5	15-25
Over 29.0	Obese	at least 7.0	15

BMI: body mass index

On the other hand, a lower amount of weight gain influences birth size. Decreased maternal weight gain is reported, decreased by approximately 2 kg from 1988 to 2002 in Japanese women, which lead to decreased average birth weight [Ueda et al., 2005]. Women who did not achieve the lower quartile value had more than twice the risk of having low-birth-weight infants. One of the possible reasons may be the restriction of weight gain excessively by health providers or the women themselves. Women may try to lose weight or restrict weight gain by dieting behaviors including restricted food intake, poor quality diet and consuming a low daily energy diet, even after they become pregnant. Additional weight gain and changes in body composition can leave many women feeling insecure about their body size and shape.

Eating attitudes and dieting practices of women due to preconceptions influence weight gain during pregnancy. It appears that women who diet habitually prior to becoming pregnant gain more weight during pregnancy and regard themselves as less accountable for their weight while pregnant [Clark and Ogden, 1999]. In a study undertaken in North Carolina, Mumford et al. [2008] found that an association between restrained eating and weight gain during pregnancy. Women with more than 19.8 kg/m^2, and a history of dieting or restrained eating gained more weight during pregnancy. In contrast, underweight women with a history of restrained eating behaviors gained less weight compared to underweight women without those behaviors.

Effective Nutritional Education

Promoting preconceptions for the health of women is a key public health strategy. Each country has special programs for improving women's health, especially for preventing NTD in offspring. The Public Health Service, including that of the U.S and Japan, recommends that all women capable of becoming pregnant consume 400μg of folic acid daily throughout childbearing years. Despite the abundance of information concerning folic acid, many women of reproductive age still are either not aware of its importance or do not value this information. The RDA guidelines have not worked effectively to appeal to the public.

Thiele et al. [2004] observed in Germany that better educated women had higher indexes of qualitatively beneficial diets than less educated women. Adolescents at universities and colleges are potentially important targets for the promotion of healthy lifestyle including physical, psychological and eating habits. However, little is known concerning nutritional and health related behavior. More effective education campaigns should be set up by health care providers to improve women's awareness. Dieticians should educate young women about careful selection of food and meal planning and preparation at the campus or through mass media.

The questions arises how pregnant women are concerned about their consumed diet, and whether pregnant women get appropriate nutrient information during their routine antenatal checkups. Bowman et al. [1998] reported that 79% of pregnant women consumed diets needing improvement. Nearly 80% of pregnant women need dietary advice [Orr and Simmons, 1979]. On the other hand, Anya et al. [2008] reported that women spend 3 minutes or less with their antenatal care providers and less than 40% had been informed or educated about diet and nutrition. These results suggest that pregnant women do not have an opportunity to get adequate and appropriate nutrition education in antenatal care. Most of them expect advice on general dietary improvements, with the remainder seeking advice on helping to promote their quality and quantity of nutritional intake. Health care providers should give individual graphs of their weight gains at each antenatal check up, having viewed as valuable sources of information on diet, nutrition, and exercise. An individualized approach is likely to have better outcomes than a standard intervention that is given to all pregnant women. A critical goal to achieve is for women to make behavior changes for good nutritional status before, during, and beyond pregnancy, which may lead to improved birth outcomes.

References

Agrahar-Murugkar, D. & Pal, P. P. (2004). Intake of nutrients and food sources of nutrients among the Khasi tribal women of India. *Nutrition*, *20*, 268-73.

Anya, S. E., Hydara, A. & Jaiteh, L. E. (2008). Antenatal care in The Gambia: missed opportunity for information, education and communication. *BMC Pregnancy Childbirth,*, *8*, 9.

Berg, C., Rosengren, A., Aires, N., Lappas, G., Toren, K., Thelle, D. & Lissner, L. (2005). Trends on overweight and obesity from 1985 to 2002 in Goteborg, West Sweden. *Int J obes (Lond)*, *29*, 916-24.

Bowman, S. A., Lino, M., Gerrior, S. A. & Basiotis, P. The healthy eating index 1994-96. Washington, DC: United States Department of Agriculture, Center for Nutrition Policy and Promotion; 1998. CNPP-5.

Carmichael, S., Abrams, B. & Selvin, S. (1997). The pattern of maternal weight gain in women with good pregnancy outcomes. *Am J Public Health*, *87*, 1984-8.

Clark, M. & Ogden, J. (1999). The impact of pregnancy on eating behaviour and aspects of weight concern. *Int J Obes Relat Metab Disord*, *23*, 18-24.

Eherenberg, H. M., Dierker, L., Milluzzi, C. & Mercer, B. M. (2003). Low maternal weight, failure to thrive in pregnancy, and adverse pregnancy outcomes. *Am J Obstet Gynecol*, *189*, 1726-30.

Ford, F. A., Mouratidou, T., Wademan, S. E. & Fraser, R. B. (2008). Effect of the introduction of "Health Start" on dietary behaviour during and after pregnancy: early results from the before and after Sheffield study. *Br J Nutr*, *19*, 1-9.

Fowles, E. R. & Murphey, C. (2009). Nutrition and mental health in early pregnancy: a pilot study. *J Midwifery Womens Health*, *54*, 73-7.

Franke, C., Verwied-Jorky, S., Campoy, C., Trak-Fellermeier, M., Decsi, T., Dolz, V. & Koletzko, B. (2008). Dietary intake of natural sources of docosahexaenoic acid and folate in pregnant women of three European cohorts. *Ann Nutr Metab*, *53*, 167-74.

Gautam, V. P., Taneja, D. K., Sharma, N., Gupta, V. K. & Ingle, G. K. (2008). Dietary aspects of pregnant women in rural areas of Northern India. *Mater Child Nutr.*, *4*, 86-94.

Helgstrand, S. & Andersen, A. M. (2005). Maternal underweight and the risk of spontaneous abortion. *Acta Obstet Gynecol Scand*, *84*, 1197-201.

ICM (Institute of Medicine). Nutrition during pregnancy: Part I Weight Gain and Part II Nutrient Supplements. Washington, DC: National Academies Press; 1990; 10-23.

Kabiru, W. & Raynor, B. D. (2004). Obstetric outcomes associated with increase in BMI category during pregnancy. *Am J Obstet Gynecol*, *191*, 928-32.

Kaiser, L. & Allen, L. H. (2008). Position of American dietetic association: nutrition and lifestyle for a healthy pregnancy outcome. *J Am Diet Assoc*, *108*, 553-61.

Kamau-Mbuthia, E. & Elmadfa, I. (2007). Diet quality of pregnant women attending an antenatal clinic in Nakuru, Kenya. *Ann Nutr Metab*, *51*, 324-30.

Knopp, R. H. (1997). Hormone mediated changes in nutrient metabolism in pregnany: a physiological basis for normal fetal development. In Adolescent Nutritional Disorders: Prevention and Treatment, Jacobsen MS, Rees JM, Golden NH, Irwin CE, Eds. New York, New York Academy of Sciences, 251-71.

Mouratidou, T., Ford, F., Prountzou, F. & Fraser, R. (2006). Dietary assessment of a population of pregnant women in Sheffield, UK. *Br J Nutr*, *96*, 929-35.

Mumford, S. L., Siega-Riz, A. M., Herring, A. & Evenson, K. R. (2008). Dietary restraint and gestational weight gain. *J Am Diet Assoc*, *108*, 1646-53.

NRCIM (National Research Council and Institute of Medicine). Influence of pregnancy weight on maternal and child Health. Workshop Report. Washington DC: National Academies Press: 2007.

Ogden, C. L., Carroll, M. D. & Flegal, K. M. (2008). High body mass index for age among US children and adolescents, 2003-2006. *JAMA*, *299*, 2442-3.

Orr, R. D. & Simmons, J. J. (1979). Nutrition care in pregnancy: the patients view 11. Perceptions, satisfaction and response to dietary advice and treatment. *J Ame Diet Asso*, *75*, 131-6.

Parker, J. D. & Abrams, B. (1992). Prenatal weight gain advice: an examination of the recent prenatal weight gain recommendations of the Institute of Medicine. *Obstet Gynecol*, *79*, 664-9.

Petrakos, G., Panagopoulos, P., Koutras, I., Kazis, A., Panagiotakos, D., Economou, A., Kanellopoulos, N., Salamalekis, E. & Zabelas, A. (2006). A comparison of the dietary and total intake of micronutrients in a group of pregnant Greek women with the Dietary Reference Intakes. *Eur J Obstet Gynecol Reprod Biol*, *127*, 166-71.

Pick, M. E., Edwards, M., Moreau, D. & Ryan, E. A. (2005). Assessment of diet quality in pregnant women using the healthy eating index. *J Am Diet Assoc*, *105*, 240-6.

Polley, B. A., Wing, R. R. & Sims, C. J. (2002). Randomized controlled trial to prevent excessive weight gain in pregnant women. *Int J Obes Relat Metab Disord*, *26*, 1494-502.

RCOG (Royal College of Obstetricians and Gynecologists), 5th October 2006 Press Releases [http://www.rcog.org.uk/news/growing-trends-maternal-obesity].

Rees, G. A., Doyle, W., Srivastava, A., Brooke, Z. M., Crawford, M. A. & Costeloe, K. L. (2005). The nutrient intakes of mothers of low birth weight babies-a comparison of ethnic groups in East London, UK. *Matern Child Nutr.*, *1*, 91-9.

Rifas-Shiman, S. L., Rich-Edwards, J. W., Willett, W. C., Kleinman, K. P., Oken, E. & Gillman, M. W. (2006). Changes in dietary intake from the first to the second trimester of pregnancy. *Paediatr Perinat Epidemiol*, *20*, 35-42.

Schieve, L. A., Cogswell, M. E. & Scanlon, K. S. (1998). Trends in pregnancy weight gain within and outside ranges recommended by the Institute of Medicine in a WIC population. *Matern Child Health J*, *2*, 111-6.

Sekiya, N., Anai, T., Matsubaara, M. & Miyazaki, F. (2007). Maternal weight gain rate in the second trimester are associated with birth weight and length of gestation. *Gynecol Obstet Invest*, *63*, 45-8.

Siega-Riz, A. M., Bodnar, L. M. & Savitz, D. A. (2002). What are pregnant women eating? Nutrient and food group differences by race. *Am J Obstet Gynecol*, *186*, 480-6.

Stotland, N. E., Cheng, Y. W., Hopkins, L. M. & Caughey, A. B. (2006). Gestational weight gain and adverse neonatal outcome among term infants. *Obstet Gynecol* 2006, *108*, 635-43.

Takimoto, H., Yoshiike, N., Katagiri, A., Ishida, H. & Abe, S. (2003). Nutritional status of pregnant and lactating women in Japan: A comparison with non-pregnant/non-lactating controls in the national nutrition survey. *J Obstet Gynecol Res*, *29*, 96-103.

Thiele, S., Mensink, G. & Beitz, R. (2004). Determinants of diet quality. *Public Health Nutr*, *7*, 29-37.

Ueda, Y., Maruo, H., Ashidaka, Y. & Honda, Y. (2005). Studies on the validity of the present criteria for optimal maternal weight gain during pregnancy: reevaluation of the change in maternal and neonatal weight occurring during the period of 15 years beginning from 1988. *Adv Obstet Gynecol*, *57*, 121-30.

Watanabe, H., Fukuoka, H., Sugiyama, T., Nagai, Y., Ogasawara, K. & Yoshiike, N. (2008). Dietary folate intake during pregnancy and birth weight in Japan. *Eur J Nutr*, *47*, 341-7.

In: Nutritional Education
Editor: Ida R. Laidyth

ISBN: 978-1-60876-078-7

Chapter 9

NUTRITION AND TUBERCULOSIS

Wing Wai Yew* and Chi Chiu Leung†*

*Chief of Service, Tuberculosis and Chest Unit, Grantham Hospital, Hong Kong, CHINA

†Consultant Chest Physician, Tuberculosis and Chest Service, Centre for Health Protection, Department of Health, Hong Kong, CHINA

ABSTRACT

Evidences are accumulating in both human and animal studies that undernutrition is associated with increased risk and severity of tuberculosis. In addition, obesity appears to protect against tuberculosis. Diabetes mellitus increases risk of tuberculosis, but poor diabetic control contributes to the bulk of such risk. In both under-nutrition and poor diabetic control, the increased risk is seen mainly in the pulmonary form of the disease, and the exact reason for relative sparing of the extrapulmonary sites remains unclear. Undernutrition has also been associated with worsened prognosis, poorer response to treatment and increased risk of relapse. Data from randomized controlled trials are scanty, as nutritional supplementation trials are often costly and difficult to implement. Micronutrients have been shown to decrease the risk of reversion of sputum culture to positivity after initial conversion, but there was no significant effect on mortality. With the putative roles of systemic inflammatory responses in tuberculosis manifestations, adjunctive corticosteroid administration treatment has been found to afford earlier and more significant body weight gain, albeit no differences in sputum bacteriological conversion and disease relapse rate. Further studies, with better study designs and serial monitoring of relevant nutritional parameters, are required to clarify the complex situation.

INTRODUCTION

Tuberculosis is commonly associated with poverty and under-nutrition in both developed and developing countries [1-4]. However, the presence of multiple potential confounders often poses considerable difficulties in delineating the exact relationship. With the often

* Corresponding Author: cc_leung@dh.gov.hk, Tel.: 852-25353864, Fax:852-29775940

chronic and insidious nature of the disease, and its multiple nutritional / metabolic effects, the exact direction of causality is generally obscure in most cross-sectional or case-control studies.

NUTRITION AND RISK OF TUBERCULOSIS

In recent years, a number of systematic reviews [5-6] have helped to summarize the previous human and animal studies on the subject. Two previous prospective studies showed higher risk of tuberculosis among underweight subjects, but the authors attributed such effect to body build [7-8]. A prospective cohort study not only reconfirmed the previous observations, but also demonstrated a substantially decreased risk of tuberculosis among those subjects who were obese at the baseline, as compared to their normal-weight counterparts [9]. The linear relationship between body mass index and tuberculosis risk suggested a close link between the nutritional status and the immune defense mechanism against the tubercle bacillus. Improving socioeconomic conditions have been associated with the decline of tuberculosis well before the advent of effective treatment in the last century [10]. Increased availability of cheaper food associated with improving socioeconomic conditions could have played a pivotal role [10]. While severe malnutrition is uncommon at peace time in developed areas nowadays, milder degree of undernutrition is probably fairly common, even among these areas, and overall nutrition status is likely to continue to have a major impact of the epidemiology of tuberculosis.

Various defects in cellular immune mechanism have also been demonstrated in animal studies, especially those on protein deprivation in the guinea pig model [11-12]. However, the interaction is likely to go beyond those related to simple nutrient deficiencies. A cholesterol-rich diet has also been shown to accelerate bacteriologic sterilization in pulmonary tuberculosis [13]. Adipose tissue is now recognized to have major endocrine functions [14]. Increasing evidence suggests that leptin differentially regulates metabolic, neuroendocrine and immune functions in human [15]. The administration of leptin in human congenital leptin deficiency has demonstrated beneficial effects on obesity, T-cell hyporesponsiveness and neuroendocrine / metabolic dysfunction [16]. Leptin-deficient ob/ob mice have been shown to be highly susceptible to pulmonary infection by *Mycobacterium tuberculosis* [17]. A better understanding of the complex interplay between the tubercle bacillus and our body is likely an important step for the discovery of new intervention targets in our battle against this long-standing enemy of humanity.

DIABETES MELLITUS

Diabetes mellitus has been well reported to be associated with increased risk of tuberculosis [18-19]. In a recent prospective cohort study in Hong Kong [20], diabetes mellitus (mainly type 2) was associated with a modest increase in risk of active, culture-confirmed and pulmonary but not extrapulmonary tuberculosis, with adjusted hazard ratios of 1.77, 1.91, 1.89 and 1.00 respectively [20]. The increased risk was observed only among diabetic patients with baseline glycosylated hemoglobin HbA1c $\geq 7\%$. They had a three-fold increase in risk in comparison with those diabetic subjects with baseline HbA1c <7%, who were not at increased risk. Substantial heterogeneity in tuberculosis risk is observed among diabetic subjects in different localities [18-21]. Apart from possible constitutional differences, including the relative proportion of type 1 and 2 diabetes, barriers of access to care and differences in diabetic control might have contributed to the ethnic differences as observed. In-vitro immune studies and skin testing among diabetic subjects have shown possible impairment of adaptive immune responses [22-25]. Similar to the effect of body mass index [8, 9], the increased risk of diabetes mellitus was relatively specific for pulmonary tuberculosis but not extrapulmonary tuberculosis. Higher prevalence of diabetes mellitus was also observed among patients with pulmonary tuberculosis as compared to those with extrapulmonary tuberculosis in a case-control study [26]. Diabetes mellitus has also been reported to modify the disease manifestation, with more frequent lower lung field involvement and cavity formation [27-28]. A close interplay between the energy metabolism and immune system could well be implicated in the relatively specific pulmonary effect of both body mass index and diabetic control.

Severity of Disease

Nutritional status has been well reported to be associated with the severity of disease [29, 30]. Again, because of the profound metabolic effect of tuberculosis, it might be difficult to be certain of the direction of causality in a cross-sectional or case-control analysis. With the increased risk of tuberculosis among the underweight, immunological effect of protein depletion in animal models, and modified disease manifestations in DM or immunocompromizing conditions, it is biological plausible that malnutrition does increase the severity of disease.

Response to Treatment

Malnutrition has also been associated with poor response to treatment [30-31]. Nutritional deficit has also been found as a negative prognostic factor in patients with miliary tuberculosis [32]. Using a nutritional risk score comprising four factors (low body mass index, hypoalbuminemia, hypocholesterolemia, and severe lymphocytopenia), the independent and major prognostic values of nutritional status on both acute respiratory failure and 90-day mortality among 56 patients with miliary tuberculosis were demonstrated. Again with the retrospective design and observational nature of this study, it might be difficult to pinpoint the exact cause and effect direction between nutrition status and tuberculosis severity / outcome.

Underweight at baseline was shown to be independently associated with relapse risk among HIV-negative tuberculosis patients in a randomized chemotherapy trial [33]. On reanalysis of the data in the same trial, the two-year relapse rates were 4.2%, 11.9, and 20.3% among those not underweight, those underweight but gaining > 5% weight at two months, and those underweight and not gaining weight, respectively, and lack of early weight gain was found to be an independent predictor of relapse in underweight tuberculosis patients (OR

2.4, P = 0.03), after controlling for other risk factors including, among others, cavity and sputum culture positivity at two months [34]. As much as 61% of relapse in that trial occurred among those ≥10% underweight at diagnosis, and 62% of these in turn occurred in those failing to gain > 5% weight in the induction phase of treatment. On the other hand, a previous study in Tanzania concluded that weight gain during tuberculosis therapy was an unreliable indicator of overall treatment response [35]. However, that study, besides including HIV-infected subjects, did not specifically examine the effect of weight change during the initial phase among patients who were underweight at diagnosis. In the absence of randomized intervention targeting at nutritional status, the question still remains regarding whether the weight gain helps to augment host defense against the mycobacterial pathogen, or just reflects successful control of the disease by the chemotherapy [36].

NUTRITIONAL SUPPLEMENTATION

Tuberculosis carries a very substantial degree of mortality, especially for the more disseminated forms of the disease in debilitated / immunocompromized host. If poor nutritional status does predispose to major complication(s) and death, specific intervention targeting at improving the nutritional status would be indicated to decrease the associated morbidity and mortality. Anti-tuberculosis drug resistance is an increasing concern globally. With our currently limited armament, it might be difficult to work out an effective regimen for those patients suffering from extensively drug-resistant tuberculosis. As only one in ten infected persons, on average, will ever develop disease in his / her lifetime, host factors appears to be critical in the defense against the tubercle bacillus. Where we are almost back to the pre-chemotherapy era, it might also be worthwhile to re-examine the role of nutritional supplementation, either alone or as adjunct to chemotherapy / surgery, in the humanitarian and active management of these unfortunate patients.

Unfortunately, systematically collected data are notably scarce in this area. In a randomized controlled trial design, micronutrients have also been shown to decrease the risk of reversion of sputum culture to positivity after initial conversion at the first month in both HIV-infected and non-infected patients, but there was no significant effect on mortality [37]. However, micronutrients benefitted HIV-uninfected subjects the most in that trial, whereas the opposite was the case in a previous trial in the same locality [38]. In anti-tuberculosis chemotherapy, bacteriological cure with absence of relapse is probably the most clinically relevant endpoint. While it is generally acceptable to use validated surrogate endpoints, such as two-month culture conversion [39] or time-to-culture conversion [40], to decrease the sample size requirement and shorten the duration of follow-up in explorative trials, caution might have to be exercised in the employment of less well characterized endpoints such as culture reversion after a single negative sputum culture at the first month. Minor variation in sputum collection technique and / or sputum processing could have produced a single negative culture when the bacillary load was lowered after a month of treatment. When multiple endpoints and subgroups were evaluated in a single trial, results should also be interpreted with care.

As tuberculosis is generally more prevalent in developing areas and nutritional supplementation is likely to show the greatest effects among those with malnourishment, an adequately powered trial will probably have to be implemented in a resources-limited area. Micronutrient deficiencies often occur in midst of global nutritional deficits. As both of them might play a role in modulating our body defense against tuberculosis, careful documentation of both overall nutritional status and specific nutrient deficiencies is desirable, so that maximal amount of information can be extracted from these often costly trials. Unfortunately, neither of the above two trials on micronutrient supplementation contained specific information on total protein-calorie intake or serial measurements of body weight or body mass index to allow clear inference.

Other Adjunctive Therapy

Systemic inflammatory responses also appear to play an important role in the development of severe complications in tuberculosis. In a study just alluded to, elevated C-reactive protein level was also shown to be an independent predictor of acute respiratory failure [32]. Poor appetite and decreased food intake may also be associated with advanced tuberculosis disease. Adjunctive corticosteroid administration during tuberculosis treatment has been found to afford earlier and more significant body weight gain, albeit no differences in sputum bacteriological conversion and disease relapse rate [41]. Such form of treatment might also merit reappraisal in clinical situations associated with heightened inflammatory responses, especially when simple dietary manipulation does not appear to result in significant improvement in the nutrition status.

Reference

[1] Barr, RG; Diez-Roux, AV; Knirsch, CA; Pablos-Mendez, A. Neighborhood poverty and the resurgence of tuberculosis in New York City 1984-1992. *Am J Public Health*, 2001, 91, 1487-93.

[2] World Health Organization. Addressing poverty in tuberculosis control. WHO/HTM/TB/2005.352. World Health Organization, 2005, Geneva.

[3] Van Lettow, M; Harries, AD; Kumwenda, JJ., et al. Micronutrient malnutrition and wasting in adults with pulmonary tuberculosis with and without HIV co-infection in Malawi. *BMC Infect. Dis.*, 2004, 4, 61.

[4] Schwenk, A; Macallan, DC. Tuberculosis, malnutrition and wasting. *Curr Opin Clin Nutr Metab Care,* 2000, 3, 285-91.

[5] Cegielski, JP; McMurray, DN. The relationship between malnutrition and tuberculosis: evidence from studies in humans and experimental animals. *Int J Tuberc Lung Dis. Mar.,* 2004, 8, 286-298.

[6] Africa's Health in 2010 project / Academy for Educational Development. Nutrition and Tuberculosis: A review of the literature and considerations for TB control programs. United States Agency for International Development 2008, Washington.

[7] Palmer, CE; Jablon, S; Edwards, PQ. Tuberculosis morbidity of young men in relation to tuberculin sensitivity and body build. *Am Rev Tuberc,* 1957, 76, 517-39.

[8] Tverdal, A. Body mass index and incidence of tuberculosis. *Eur J Respir Dis.,* 1986, 69, 355-62.

[9] Leung, CC; Lam, TH; Chan, WM., et al. Lower risk of tuberculosis in obesity. *Arch Intern Med.,* 2007, 167, 1297-304.

[10] Fairchild, AL; Oppenheimer, GM. Public health nihilism vs pragmatism: history, politics, and the control of tuberculosis. *Am J Public Health.*, 1998, 88, 1105-17.

[11] Dai, G; McMurray, DN. Altered cytokine production and impaired antimycobacterial immunity in protein malnourished guinea pigs. *Infect Immun,* 1998, 66, 3562–3568.

[12] Mainali, ES; McMurray, DN. Adoptive transfer of resistance to pulmonary tuberculosis in guinea pigs is altered by protein deficiency. *Nutr Res.,* 1998, 118, 309–317.

[13] Perez-Guzman, C; Vargas, MH; Quinonez, F; Bazavilvazo, N; Aguilar, A. A cholesterol-rich diet accelerates bacteriologic sterilization in pulmonary tuberculosis. *Chest*, 2005, 127, 643-51.

[14] Rondinone, CM. Adipocyte-derived hormones, cytokines, and mediators. *Endocrine*, 2006, 29, 81-90.

[15] Chan, JL; Matarese, G; Shetty, GK., et al. Differential regulation of metabolic, neuroendocrine, and immune function by leptin in humans. *Proc Natl Acad Sci USA.,* 2006, 103, 8481-6.

[16] Farooqi, IS; Matarese, G; Lord, GM., et al. Beneficial effects of leptin on obesity, T cell hyporesponsiveness, and neuroendocrine/metabolic dysfunction of human congenital leptin deficiency. *J Clin Invest,* 2002, 110, 1093-103.

[17] Wieland, CW; Florquin, S; Chan, ED., et al. Pulmonary Mycobacterium tuberculosis infection in leptin-deficient ob/ob mice. *Int Immunol,* 2005, 17, 1399-408.

[18] Kim, SJ; Hong, YP; Lew, WJ., et al. Incidence of pulmonary tuberculosis among diabetics. *Tuber Lung Dis*., 1995, 76, 529–33.

[19] Coker, R; McKee, M; Atun, R., et al. Risk factors for pulmonary tuberculosis in Russia: case-control study. *BMJ*, 2006, 332, 85-7.

[20] Leung, CC; Lam, TH; Chan, WM., et al. Diabetic Control and Risk of Tuberculosis: A Cohort Study. *Am J Epidemiol*, 2008, 167, 1486-94.

[21] Olmos, P; Donoso, J; Rojas, N., et al. Tuberculosis and diabetes mellitus: a longitudinal-retrospective study in a teaching hospital. *Rev Med Chil.*, 1989, 117, 979-83.

[22] Casey, JI; Heeter, BJ; Klyshevich, KA. Impaired response of lymphocytes of diabetic subjects to antigen of Staphylococcus aureus. *J Infect Dis*., 1977, 136, 495–501.

[23] Eibl, N; Spatz, M; Fischer, GF., et al. Impaired primary immune response in type-1 diabetes: results from a controlled vaccination study. *Clin Immunol*, 2002, 103, 249–259.

[24] Pozzilli, P; Pagani, S; Arduini, P., et al. In vivo determination of cell mediated immune response in diabetic patients using a multiple intradermal antigen dispenser. *Diabetes Res*., 1987, 6, 5–8

[25] Spatz, M; Eibl, N; Hink, S., et al. Impaired primary immune response in type-1 diabetes. Functional impairment at the level of APCs and T-cells. *Cell Immunol,* 2003, 221, 15–26.

[26] Antony, SJ; Harrell, V; Christie, JD., et al. Clinical differences between pulmonary and extrapulmonary tuberculosis: a 5-year retrospective study. *J Natl Med Assoc.,* 1995, 87, 187-92.

[27] Perez-Guzman, C; Torres-Cruz, A; Villarreal-Velarde, H., et al. Atypical radiological images of pulmonary tuberculosis in 192 diabetic patients: a comparative study. Int *J Tuberc Lung Dis*., 2001, 5, 455-61.

[28] Shaikh, MA; Singla, R; Khan, NB., et al. Does diabetes alter the radiological presentation of pulmonary tuberculosis. *Saudi Med J.,* 2003, 24, 278-81.

[29] Van Lettow, M; Kumwenda, JJ; Harries, AD., et al. Malnutrition and the severity of lung disease in adults with pulmonary tuberculosis in Malawi. *Int J Tuberc Lung Dis.,* 2004, 8, 211-7.

[30] Zachariah, R; Spielmann, MP; Harries, AD; Salaniponi, FM. Moderate to severe malnutrition in patients with tuberculosis is a risk factor associated with early death. *Tran R Soc Trop Med Hyg.,* 2002, 96, 291-4.

[31] Harries, AD; Nkhoma, WA; Thompson, PJ; Nyangulu, DS; Wirima, JJ. Nutritional status in Malawian patients with pulmonary tuberculosis and response to chemotherapy. Eur *J Clin Nutr.,* 1988, 42, 445-50.

[32] Kim, DK; Kim, HJ; Kwon, SY; et al. Nutritional deficit as a negative prognostic factor in patients with miliary tuberculosis. *Eur Respir J.,* 2008, 32, 1031-6.

[33] Benator, D; Bhattacharya, M; Bozeman, L., et al. Tuberculosis Trials Consortium. Rifapentine and isoniazid once a week versus rifampicin and isoniazid twice a week for treatment of drug-susceptible pulmonary tuberculosis in HIV-negative patients: a randomized clinical trial. *Lancet*, 2002, 360, 528 – 534.

[34] Khan, A; Sterling, TR; Reves, R; Vernon, A; Horsburgh, CR. Tuberculosis Trials Consortium. Lack of weight gain and relapse risk in a large tuberculosis treatment trial. *Am J Respir Crit Care Med.,* 2006, 174, 344-8

[35] Kennedy, N; Ramsay, A; Uiso, L; Gutmann, J; Ngowi, FI; Gillespie, SH. Nutritional status and weight gain in patients with pulmonary tuberculosis in Tanzania. *Trans R Soc Trop Med Hyg.,* 1996, 90, 162 – 166.

[36] Yew, WW; Leung, CC. Prognostic significance of early weight gain in underweight patients with tuberculosis. Am *J Respir Crit Care Med*., 2006, 174, 236-7.

[37] Villamor, E; Mugusi, F; Urassa, W., et al. A Trial of the Effect of Micronutrient Supplementation on Treatment Outcome, T Cell Counts, Morbidity, and Mortality in Adults with Pulmonary Tuberculosis. *J Infect Dis*., 2008, 197, 1499-1505

[38] Range, N; Changalucha, J; Krarup, H; Magnussen, P; Andersen, AB; Friis, H. The effect of multi-vitamin/mineral supplementation on mortality during treatment of pulmonary tuberculosis: a randomised two-by-two factorial trial in Mwanza, Tanzania. *Br J Nutr.,* 2006, 95, 762-70.

[39] Mitchison, DA. Assessment of new sterilizing drugs for treating pulmonary tuberculosis by culture at 2 months. *Am Rev Respir Dis*., 1993, 147, 1062-1063.

[40] Holtz, TH; Sternberg, M; Kammerer, S., et al. Time to sputum culture conversion in multidrug-resistant tuberculosis: predictors and relationship to treatment outcome. *Ann Intern Med*., 2006, 144, 650-9.

[41] Bilaceroglu, S; Perim, K; Buyuksirin, M; Celikten, E. Prednisolone: a beneficial and safe adjunct to anti-tuberculous treatment? A randomized controlled trial. Int *J Tuberc Lung Dis*., 1999, 3, 47–54

In: Nutritional Education
Editor: Ida R. Laidyth

ISBN: 978-1-60876-078-7

Chapter 10

EFFECTIVENESS OF EDUCATIONAL PROGRAMS AIMED AT PROMOTING HEALTHY LIFESTYLE FOR OBESITY PREVENTION AMONG CHILDREN*

A. Tripodi[1], S. Severi[1], S. Midili[1] and A.V. Ciardullo[2]

[1] Food Hygiene and Nutrition Service,
Department of Public Health, AUSL Modena, Italy

[2] Diabetes Unit, Hospital Department of Internal Medicine,
AUSL Modena, Italy

ABSTRACT

The rapid and steady rise in the incidence of obesity during childhood and adolescence in all western countries, and also the developing world, has reached such levels that experts now talk of "an obesity epidemic". Strategies therefore need to be carried out swiftly to promote a healthy diet and lifestyle.

The World Health Organization's report "Global strategy on diet, physical activity and health" stresses the importance of implementing these policies during childhood if they are to be effective, and emphasies the role of public authorities and various sectors of the local community. Unfortunately, reports show that up till now, many strategies implemented at an early age have failed to produce significant long-term changes in daily eating and exercise habits. In many cases, the failure of such interventions can be linked to an inadequate knowledge of various important factors, such as the behaviour, attitudes and habits of the children involved in the study, as well as the socio-economic, urbanistic and geographic aspects of the community where they live.

Content: Nutritional monitoring programmes which provide local information (or at least regional) make it possible to collect the necessary data for planning community health strategies and to evaluate the results. Data regarding children's eating and physical activity habits, their awareness of nutrition, the desired educational approach, the main sources of information used, along with the extent of mass-media influence and

* A version of this chapter was also published in Child Nutrition Research Advances, edited by Laura V. Carter, Nova Science Publishers. It was submitted for appropriate modifications in an effort to encourage wider dissemination of research

advertising, can be obtained from primary schools, using suitably designed and administered questionnaires. Family members can provide the same information about pre-school children, along with more general information about family structure, socio-economic conditions, their reaction to the principle of "healthy eating" and habits regarding the child's likes and dislikes. This information, together with essential requisites for efficient healthy eating and physical exercise strategy, are taken from authoritative reviews (schools provide an excellent site for policy implementation, multidimensional approach, few and easily understood messages, definition of practical solutions, long-term projects, involvement of all community partners). These aspects will be looked at in more detail in the article through the direct experience of Nutritional Monitoring and the planning and implementation of strategies targeted at preventing childhood obesity.

Conclusion: Awareness of the population's eating and physical activity habits is essential for carrying out educational policies. Long-term educational projects, when the community's "leading players" take an active role, seem to help establish healthy eating and physical activity habits right from childhood.

INTRODUCTION

Burden of Obesity

A healthy lifestyle does improve people's health at each age-class.

In a recent report, WHO [1] showed the great burden of mortality, morbidity and disabling attributable to chronic disease (i.e., cardiovascular diseases, cancer, type 2 diabetes, obesity, osteoporosis, etc.) affecting both developed and poor countries worldwide.

Risk factors for chronic diseases are of two types: *genetic risk factors* that are not modifiable but whose expression is affected by socio-environmental conditions, and *behavioural and environmental risk factors* that are modifiable and should be the object of health promotion and primary disease prevention.

Most important risk factors for chronic disease are high blood pressure, high plasma lipids, cigarette smoking, overweight/obesity, sedentariness, and low intake of fruit and vegetables. Their relationship with eating habits and physical activity is self-evident.

Diet is a key health determinant. In particular, we have to pay attention to overfeeding and the prevention of overweight/obesity thus preventing chronic diseases both through weight loss and metabolic amelioration (e.g., by reducing insulin-resistance) [2].

The prevalence of overweight and obesity rapidly increased worldwide as a "global epidemic" [3-7]. Body mass index (BMI) (kg/m^2) is commonly used to define overweight and obesity in clinical and epidemiologic studies because it correlates well with more accurate measures of body fat, and its measurement is reliable and non-intrusive [8-10]. The definition of international standards for BMI - also for children and adolescents [11] - favoured international comparisons.

In the last three decades the prevalence of obesity in USA has doubled, affecting about 1/3 of the general populaton [12, 13]. In some Latin American countries, globalisation has changed the face of obesity. In Mexico and Brazil, for example, where overweight used to be a sign of wealth, it now often marks poverty. While the upper class can choose to adopt a healthy lifestyle, the poor have fewer food choices and more limited access to nutrition education. [14]. Obesity is relatively common in Europe, especially among women of South and East-Europe. The prevalence of obesity ranges from 10% to 25% across Europe. In the last decade, the incidence of obesity in Europe showed a 10-40% increment (minimum in France and maximum in Greece and UK) [15]. The very great increment did occur in UK with a three-fold prevalence since 1980.

Prevalence of obesity among children and adolescents is of great interest. Obesity is less associated with morbidity in infancy and adolescence [16] but is a strong precursor of obesity-related morbidity in adulthood [17-21]. The probability of an obese child to be an obese adult increases, if one or both the parents are overweight [22]. In terms of critical periods to develop obesity, some studies identify three peaks: 1 years, 5-6 years, and puberty period [23-25]. The age of 5-6 years is also particularly interesting as it falls within the period in which the so-called "adiposity rebound" occurs: i.e. the time at which there is a physiological increase in BMI following the decrease that takes place after the first year of life. The type and timing of the adiposity rebound may be a marker of the development of overweight in children [25,26].

Some authors underline a possible etiological role of nutritional disorders since prenatal era [23, 27].

In USA, the prevalence of obesity among children and adolescents has doubled in the past 2 decades [28]. The prevalence of overweight in children (6-9 years) and adolescents (10-18 years) tripled in Brazil from 1974 to 1997, and increased by one-fifth in China from 1991 to 1997 [29]. A drastic increase in overweight and obesity has also been observed in Australia [30] and other countries [31].

A recent joint report of the International Obesity Taskforce (IOTF) and the European Association for the Study of Obesity (EASO) show similar data on infant population in Europe (Figure 1) [33].

Bellizzi et al. [32] showed a prevalence of overweight and obesity at 15 years of age ranging from 5.8% (Dutch males) to 22.8% (Italian males).

As shown in table 1, using the international standards by IOTF [11] in Italy the prevalence of overweight among children and adolescents range from 16.5% to 19.8%, and obesity range from 6.4% to 8.9% [34-38]. The prevalence of overweight and obesity seems to be lower in Italian surveys that utilise age-adjusted national standards by Cacciari et al. [41].

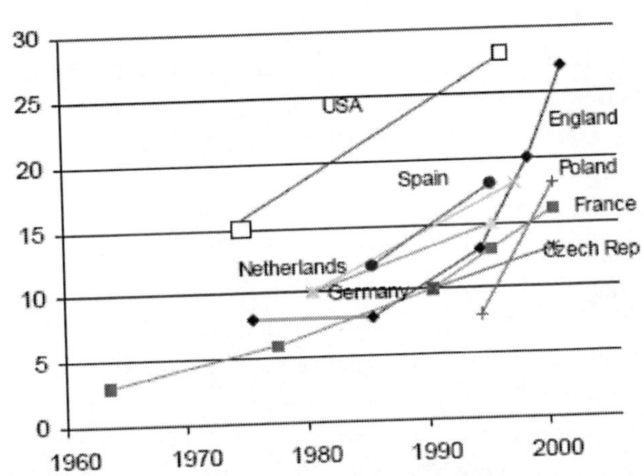

Figure 1. Trends of overweight among 5-11 years old children in Europe and USA; [From ref. 33].

Table 1. Prevalence of overweight and obesity in Italian children and adolescents, using international BMI cut-off points (11)

Source	Italy areas	Age Goup Years	Prevalence (%)	
			Overweight	Obesity
Lobstein et al (34)	Several provinces (North, Central, South Italy)	7-11	36.0*	
Celi et al (36)	Provinces of Perugia, Terni, Rieti (Central Italy)	3-17	19.9	6.4
Maffeis et al (37)	City of Verona (North Italy) City of Messina (South Italy)	2-6	16.6	8.0
Marras et al (35)	Southern Sardinia (South Italy)	6-12	18.5	7.8
Albertini et al (38)	Emilia-Romagna region (Central-North Italy)	6-9	18.7	8.9

* Excess weight (overweight + obesity).

Anyway, irrespective of the standards used there is agree about the fact that the major problem of overweight is in range 6-13 years of age, especially among males. According to a recent multicentric national survey by the Italian National Institute of Nutrition (INRAN) (unpublished data) the Italia region with the higher rate of overweight is Campania (Neaples district) in South-Italy (36%), and the lower one is Valle d'Aosta (Mont Blanc district) in North-Italy (14%). In general, in Italy there is evidence of a North-South gradient [37, 41, 42].

Risk Factors for Infant Obesity

Several studies showed that genetic background is an important determinant of susceptibility to obesity. Estimate of heritability is 50% [43]. However, interactions between genetic, psychological, biological, socio-cultural, and environmental factors are evident in childhood obesity [27, 44]. These last factors are crucial to allow dietary choices of high nutritional quality, to access healthy food, to have greater information on healthy lifestyles or to be involved in health promotion campaigns, and to defeat sedentariness.

In industrialised societies, adults with a medium-low level of education and less qualified occupations are not only more at risk of overweight and obesity themselves [45], but their influence on their family's diet and lifestyle also leads to a greater risk of obesity for their children [40,46]. Previous studies have showed that children with low family incomes and lower cognitive stimulation are at risk to develop obesity [47,48]. Moreover, children whose parents are not employed or non-professional are significantly more obese as compared with children whose parents are executives/managers [47].

Several studies reported that children and adolescents of lower socioeconomic status eat less vegetables and fruit [49,50]. One possible explanation is that lower levels of education and poorer access to relevant information reduce the capacity to make informed and healthy choices. Others suggest that the highest cost of healthier diets may contribute to the obesity epidemic, especially among the lower-income groups [51]. Rose et al, reported, in the United States, that food-insecure individuals may be at risk of overweight because they can only afford to consume food witch tend to be energy dense [52].

Also physical exercise is important in the prevention of weight gain, through the impact on energy balance, but it also appears to have an independent effect on body and mind wellness of people [53, 54].

Excess body weight results from energy intake in excess of expenditure. People in industrialized countries are expending less energy in activities of daily living, and at work [55]. The same is for infant age, in fact children spend more and more time in sedentary activities such as playing video games, television watching and personal computing [2].

It has been reported that lifestyle approaches to physical activity (walking, climbing staircases, parking far from the working place, etc) may result in body weight changes and fitness improvement that are similar to what is observed with sporting exercise [56]. In addition, reduced sedentary activity is an achievable goal, whereas the institution of structured intervention after sedentary life is not likely to be a maintainable solution [57].

Currently, it is suggested that adults have at least 30 min/d of moderate-intensity physical activity to gain significant improvements in health [2, 53], up to 60 min/d if weight loss is needed [58].

Current international guidelines for children and adolescents recommend at least 60 min/d of moderate-intense daily exercise [59].

Another important environmental risk factor for excess body weight is the television (TV) watching.

In an interesting longitudinal study carried out in 9-14 year hold children, Berkey et al (60) showed that after 1 year of follow-up, increases in BMI were higher in both boys and girls with more hours of TV/videos/games. The authors estimate a 0.2 kg/m^2 increase in BMI per year of TV/videos/games. Furthermore, children watching 4 or more hours of television every day are more overweight than those who watch less than 2 hours per day [61].

TV watching should be considered a marker of sedentariness. A recent study in adolescents (62), showed that TV viewing is not related to changes in leisure-time moderate/vigorous physical activity, and a positive relationship was observed between changes in total sedentary behaviour and changes in leisure-time moderate/vigorous physical activity,. These data have been confirmed by others [61]. The authors conclude that TV viewing and physical activity are separate constructs and that simply restricted television watching may not be effective in increasing physical activity.

Public health programs should promote either TV watching reduction and physical activity increase.

TV might also affect overweight through dietary intake modifications. In the Western world about 20-25% of daily energy is consumed in front of the television [63]. First, children tend to have snacks while viewing TV [63]. Second, TV advertising tends to promote consumption of foods and beverages higher in energy density, [64, 65] and TV watching favours eating habits in children, resulting in higher energy intake [66].

Effectiveness of the Interventions

Several review articles on prevention of children and adolescents overweight and obesity have been published [67-70].

The key elements of an effective intervention aimed at the prevention of infant obesity are shown in table 2.

Table 2. Key elements of interventions to prevent infant obesity

1	School is the best setting
2	Multidimensional interventions
3	Simple, direct and few messages
4	Teachers are the preferred health educator
5	Favour a direct involvement of the children and adolescents
6	Practical solutions and examples are needed
7	Programs have to promote the consumption of healthy snacks
8	Family partnership is needed
9	Permanent interventions are needed
10	It is necessary to address extra-school time and habits

Schools are an ideal environment for such programs and the evidence is clear that overweight risk factor and fitness can be positively implemented in this setting. Moreover, schools are the only setting where children and adolescents from any socio-economic level are bought together for many hours a week for several years.

It is extremely important to involve stakeholders and target people in the development of programs to build acceptance by children, families and communities.

Multi-strategic and multifaceted educational and environmental interventions to prevent obesity are necessary. Successful programs use many elements such as behavioural curricula implementation, physical activity promotion in and out of school, improving access to healthy food choices, school food service control, parental involvement/education, and reduction of TV watching, videotapes and videogames use. Mono-disciplinary interventions are not useful, except those aimed at limiting television viewing among children [68]. In fact, Robinson showed - among 8-10 year-old children – a real improvement in anthropometrics (BMI, triceps skin-fold thickness and waist circumference) in the intervention group that had a significant decrease of television watching as compared with control group [71]. In general, TV watching seems to be the most modifiable behaviour, followed by physical activity and nutrition behaviours.

Childhood overweight and obesity intervention may be applied a large scale and are sustainable.

Nutrition specialists may improve the quality of interventions, but high economic resources are needed. Nevertheless, a great deal of effective intervention on behaviour changes have been implemented utilizing teachers with additional training. This seems to be the most feasible and practical approach [72]. In particular, the promotion of healthy snacks at school – especially fruit and vegetables - is of crucial relevance. Studies on this topic are summarised in a recent literature review [73]. Most interventions were effective to increase the daily intake of fruit and vegetables, at least in the short term, but they failed to reach the recommended 5-a-day portions [73, 74]. A higher taste preferences for fruit than for vegetables was seen, and this might partly be due to innate predispositions of humans for sweet than for bitter tastes, and vegetable often have somewhat bitter taste. Female children showed higher fruit and vegetables consumption than males. The habit to have fruit in the morning snack is crucial, and have influence on total daily food intake. A too caloric snack in the morning determines higher plenty at lunch thus favouring an excess calorie intake at the snack in the afternoon. These behaviours may induce overweight in the children [75].

The majority of published studies are short term, i.e. duration less than 1 year [67-70].

Health programs have be sustained in the long run. Systematic reviews generally include only randomised control trials (RCT). But randomisation is difficult to be done in health promotion, especially when the target is general population [72]. Health promotion interventions are often multifaceted and each component of the intervention may be synergist or enabling with every other. In very long term interventions is difficult to control for known and unknown confounders. Other authors [67, 68] consider larger inclusion criteria of the studies to address these aspects.

However, further research is required to understand the merits of the various forms and settings in which interventions are delivered to be effective.

Our Work: The Community Programs

In the last 5 years, Italian Health authorities paid increasing attention to overweight and obesity prevention among children and adolescents. For this reason, the last two National Health Plans gave a central role to the promotion of healthy lifestyles among the general population in order to prevent obesity and related chronic disease, especially cardiovascular diseases.

International recommendations [53] focused on the need to avoid the fragmentation of the interventions and to define different roles of local, regional and national health systems. Health governmental organisations has to create partnerships with producers and traders to promote the diffusion of healthy food, especially foods low in refined sugars and calories; to put the rules of food advertising on mass-media; to modify scholar curricula introducing health education and increasing the hours of physical exercise.

We lack of a nutritional surveillance agency at a national level able to monitor time-trends of overweight and obesity.

At a regional and local level, policy and institutional programs for the promotion of healthy lifestyles among the general and scholar population are developing such as safe dedicate tracks to let pupils walking or cycling for going to school, more urban green, or indoor implants to increase sporting. In other words, we need a continue struggle against the ”obesogenic environment”.

Our methodology is defined in the Local Health Plan, a real pact between the stakeholders - Institutions, citizens and enterprise – i.e., all the actors involved as partners in gaining the health targets.

On these basis, we undergo “Community programs” for the promotion of healthy lifestyles. We address our interventions to homogenous groups in the community in order to give the participants a confirmation of their good practices, to favour the continuity of interventions over time, and to promote a virtuous cycle of health promotion.

The Community Programs

Our interventions are based on social cognitive theory [76]. Our aim is (i) to promote knowledge for healthy choices about eating and exercise habits, (ii) to increase children's and adults' self-awareness on the effectiveness of healthy changes. The collective effectiveness may be perceived in a health-oriented community. In a Community Program, each member is able to ameliorate his own and others' health thus indirectly affecting the "obesity epidemic" by improving capabilities and autonomy as well as social participation of parents and children [77]. These programs are also based on the financing of community authorities.

Children are the priority population for interventions [70, 78]. In fact, childhood is the critical age for effective health promotion [23-25], since children are open-mind and are prone to change their habits. Furthermore, healthy habits acquired in childhood are more likely to be held in adulthood [79].

Our interventions are mainly targeted to students (3-14 years-old) because in our region the school frequency is mandatory at this age.

Setting Analysis

We work in Modena province that counts about 665.000 inhabitants.

Preventing overweight and obesity requires understanding of dietary habits and the factors affecting children and their families' nutritional choices and behaviours and monitoring the "obesogenic environment" in which children live. The acquisition of these data is the task of nutritional surveillance [80].

In the last decade, large scale works in nutritional consumptions and habits have been conducted in Italy by the Italian National Institute of Food and Nutritional Research (INRAN) and the Italian National Institute of Statistics (ISTAT).

At a local level, we did analyse our infants and their families [38,40]. Our findings gave light to design subsequent health interventions. About a quarter of 6 years-old children and about a third of 9 years-old children are overweight showing an increasing trend with age. As to the children's eating habits, the majority of them have a regular Italian breakfast with low rates of night snacks. This feature seems to exclude the frequent meals as cause of infant obesity [75]. As expected we found a low intake of fruit and vegetables: 30% of 6 years-old children did not have vegetable at lunch or dinners, and 67% of them had fruit at lunch and 50% at dinner. Very low was the fish consumption.

Nine years-old children showed a good knowledge of the Mediterranean diet. They showed the wish to learn more about nutrition through active lessons such as school laboratories, small farms visits, multimedia tools, etc. Instead, they showed a low level of physical activity.

We did analyse concurrent interventions both from dietary enterprise, press and health institutions in order to counteract conflicting messages. Fortunately, in our culture there is a general distrust towards advertising. The main sources of nutritional information are public NHS physicians and dieticians followed by newspapers/magazines, TV/radio, and pack/label. (figure 2).

The socio-economic and educational level of the parents is high (60% of them has high school or degree), so families are potentially receptive to health promotion interventions.

We focused our interventions on the promotion of higher daily intake of fruit and vegetables, physical exercise and children's criticism towards TV and media advertising. The main barriers for parents to healthy dietary habits were busy daily activities and working timetable (table 3).

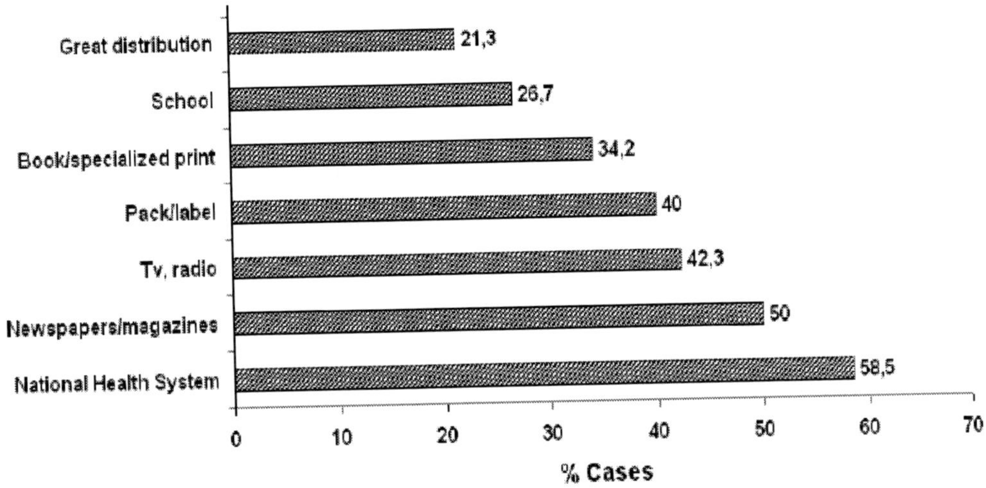

Figure 2. Children aged 6-years. The sources of parents' nutrition information (From ref. 38).

Table 3. Children aged 6-years. The main barriers for parents to healthy dietary habits (From ref. 40)

Rank		% of responses
1	Busy daily activities	20.3
2	Working timetable	16.5
3	Taste preferences	14.1
4	More time needed to cook healthy food	8.9
5	Healthy food is expensive	8.0
6	Healthy food is less palatable	6.0
7	Lack of willpower	4.8
8	Low culinary skills	4.8
9	Low knowledge on healthy food	3.6
10	Varying experts' opinion	3.4
11	Healthy food is more perishable	2.8
12	Healthy food is very far from our feeding style	2.8
13	Unwilling to change	1.4
14	None	2.4

For this reason, information materials for families contained very few key messages presented in friendly and funny styles.

Other Institutions are involved in health promotion: the Italian Minister of Health, the Regional Agriculture Councillorship, the Province Agriculture Councillorship, the Agriculturist representatives, the great distribution.

Finally, we have a regular school food service control with appropriate daily scholar menus designed by our dieticians according to the INRAN's recommendations. Furthermore, in the last two years we educated the operators of the school catering to ameliorate the quality of food and thier preparation and conservation.

We summarised the main factors affecting children's eating and exercise habits in figure 3.

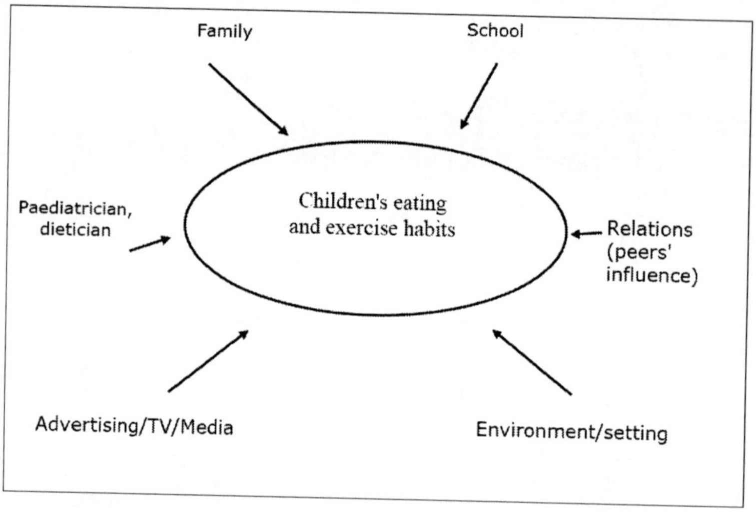

Figure 3. Factors affecting children's eating and exercise habits.

Working Phase

Our program is based on the following general criterions:

- the opportunity to implement scholar plans to prevent obesity and overweight. School is the ideal setting to carry on effective actions;
- the knowledge of the central role of diet, nutrition and physical exercise in the prevention of chronic diseases;
- the utilisation of simple and easy messages as the elective tool to health promotion among general population. Our health promotion campaign's first aim is to underline to positive and funny habits related to healthy lifestyles;
- to pay attention to the contribution of 'expert' citizens such as the teachers;
- long term programming and continuity;
- factual involvement of local institutions with a coordinating role and with structural (e.g. cycle tracks) or organisational competences (e.g. easy access to sport buildings);
- partnership with stakeholders (e.g. Agriculture Councillorships, great distribution enterprises, sport clubs);
- directness of the whole program at all communication levels (multimedia, leaflets, web, leisure activities).

We promote healthy dietary habits in the primary school since 2003. By now, we reached about 2.600 children and adolescents.

Our permanent program is formed by:

- an educational course for the teachers
- the production and dissemination of the information materials for educational scholar sessions lead by the teachers with the full involvement of the students' families
- a prized competition on the target topics, i.e. healthy nutrition and regular exercise

1. The *educational course* for the teachers is aimed at: (i) creating a network of school and health operators, (ii) sharing a basic platform of values and scopes and an effective partnership on the two main topics: nutrition and exercise; (iii) sharing knowledge and tools to implement the program at school according to a multidisciplinary approach; (iv) validating information and educational tools through small groups sessions.

The core knowledge is represented by the following issues: (i) Psychogical aspects of nutrition and feeding, (ii) Food and oral hygiene; (iii) Critical appraisal of literature evidences and guidelines; (iv) Education on the characteristics of the Mediterranean Diet [81, 82]; (v) Analysis of current not evidence based eating patterns; (vi) Advertising's role and techniques; (vii) Basis and educational techniques to promote exercise; (viii) Shared key messages.

2. The *production and dissemination of the information materials for educational scholar sessions* is realised during the educational course together with the participant teachers. The implementation and didactical strategy is self-defined by the teachers themselves: frontal lessons, class laboratories, sample healthy snacks consumed in class, the review of food allowed for classroom events, innovative exercise sessions.

As planned during the base course, teachers have to engage partnership with the territorial stakeholders from social (e.g. sport clubs) and industrial word (great distribution, dietary factories, etc.). The main objective of the educational pathway is to promote the daily consumption of fruit and vegetables [73, 83-86] among 3-7 years-old children whereas the main target is the promotion of regular daily exercise [53] among 8-14 years-old subjects. Teachers are supplied with the information materials produced by our service. The whole campaign has a 'clever little fox' named 'Boy-Fox' as testimonial (figure 4). We used a '*mascotte*' in order to be winning both for pupils and their families and mainly to give a familiar logo to the education program. Parents are informed by the school materials of the campaign's issues and they are invited to be in line with our contents about healthy eating and exercise. At the beginning of the course we propose to the teachers, students and their parents to undersign the "pact for healthy nutrition and exercise" in which the objectives and contents of the campaign are clearly stated. This represents a formal responsibility assumption.

3. The *prized competition* is a sort of 'lotto' on the target topics addressed to the students and their parents.

The lotto is addressed to all the schools in the district and asks the students to produce graphs, paints, poems, etc., on the target topics. A specific 'jury', formed by school and health operators, will assign the prizes to the best works. The prizes are some quotes of money to be used from the winner schools to buy educational materials and multimedia.

The community interventions are carried out in some municipalities counting 55.800 inhabitants. In these districts task forces among schools and the local community were created. The workshop included public authorities, local representative, mass catering, sport clubs, healthcare organisations, paediatricians and food retailers. All together with the aim of supporting through school district wellness policies and an environment that promotes access to a healthy lifestyle. In particular, we favour interventions to promote breastfeeding, to consume more vegetables and fruit at day, to increasing the levels of physical activity among children through more sport opportunities, to encouraging "the walking school bus".

The evaluation of these interventions should be concluded in a few years. Preliminarily, we have seen some improvements in fruit (figure 5) and vegetables (figure 6) daily intake during school meals.

In line with literature findings [73], we too found greater improvements in fruit than vegetables consumption.

We actually are trying to extend the whole program to the entire province area.

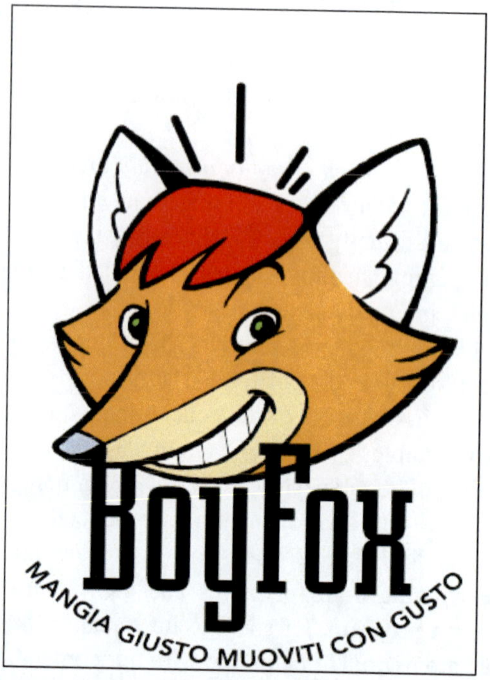

Figure 4. BoyFox, the program *mascotte* [tr. Eat right, enjoy moving].

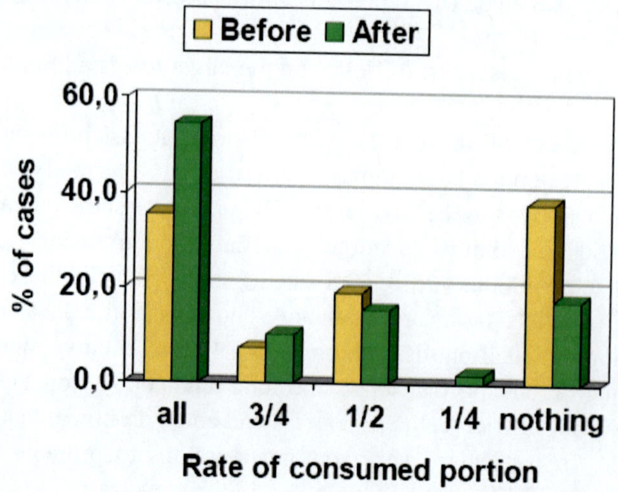

Figure 5. Improvement of fruit (apple) intake at school among children participating to the program.

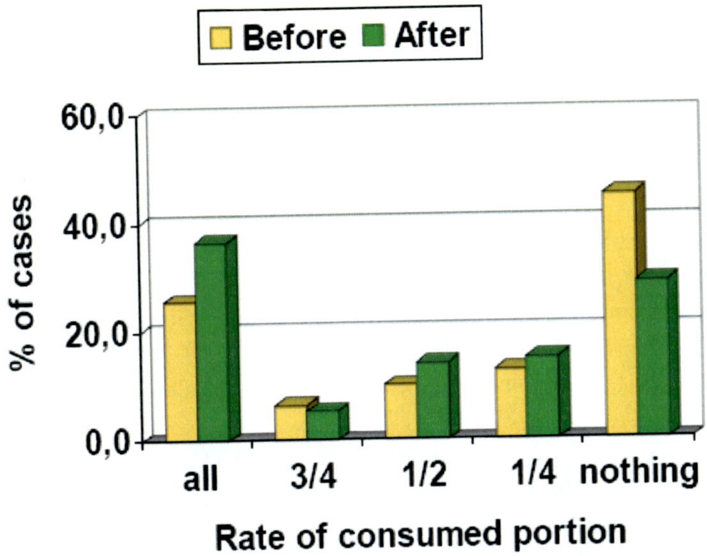

Figure 6. Improvement of vegetable (salad) intake at school among children participating to the program.

CONCLUSION

Preventive strategies should consider critical periods of early onset of obesity. It has been proposed that prevention of pediatric obesity may be the only effective treatment of adult obesity. School play a key role in the promotion of lifelong healthy habits in children. In fact, schools have many opportunities to engage children in physical activity and healthy eating and to reinforce healthy diet and physical activity messages. Every intervention at school level will need to be matched by changes in the social and cultural context so that the benefits can be sustained and enhanced. So, public health strategies to prevent obesity should begin with schools and extend to entire community. This may improve the cost-effective of the interventions [87].

REFERENCES

[1] World Health Organization – Executive Board (2003). Integrated prevention of noncommunicable disease. Available at: *http://www.who.int/chp/about/integrated_cd/en/print.html.* Accessed March 5, 2007.

[2] World Health Organization. (2003). *Diet, Nutrition and the Prevention of Chronic Diseases.* Technical Report Series, n° 916.

[3] Kuczmarski, R. J, Flegal, K. M, Campbell, S. M, & Johnson, C. L (1994). Increasing prevalence of overweight among US adults. The National Health and Nutrition Examination Surveys, 1960 to 1991. *JAMA, 272*, 205-21

[4] International Obesity Taskforce. Available at: *http://www.iotf.org*. Accessed March 7, 2007.

[5] Kimm, S. Y. & Obarzanek, E (2002): Childwood obesity: a new pandemic of the new millennium. *Pediatrics, 110*, 1003-1007:

[6] Lissau, I., Overpech, M. D., Ruan, J., Due, P., Holstein, B. E, & Hediger, M. L. (2004). Body mass index and overweight in adolescents in 13 european countries, Israel, and the United States. *Arch. Pediatr. Adolesc. Med, 158*, 27-33.

[7] International Obesity Taskforce (2005). Available at: *http://ec.europa.eu/health/ph_determinants/life_style/nutrition/documents/iotf_en.pdf*. Accessed March 7, 2007.

[8] Ellis, K. J., Abrams, S. A. & Wong, W. W. (1999). Monitoring childhood obesity: assessment of the weigt/height index. *Am. J. Epidemiol, 150 (9),* 939-946.

[9] Bellizzi, M. C. & Dietz, W. H. (1999). Workshop on childhood obesity: summary of the discussion. *Am. J. Clin. Nutr, 70 (1),* 173S-175S.

[10] Pietrobelli, A., Faith. M. S., Allison, D. B., Gallagher, D., Chiumello, G. & Heymsfield, S. B. (1998). Body mass index as a measure of adiposity among children and adolescents: a validation study. *J. Pediatr, 132*, 204 –210

[11] Cole, T. J., Bellizzi, M. C., Flegal, K. M. & Dietz, W. H (2000): Establishing a standard definition for child overweight and obesity worldwide: international survey. *BMJ, 320*, 1240-1247.

[12] Flegal, K. M., Carroll, M. D, Ogden, C. L. & Johnson, C. L.. (2002). Prevalence and trends in obesity among US adults, 1999-2000. *JAMA, 288,* 1723-7.

[13] Ogden, C. L, Carroll, M. D, Curtin, L. R, McDowell, M. A, Tabak, C. J, & Flegal, K. M. (2006). Prevalence of overweight and obesity in the United States, 1999-2004. *JAMA, 295,* 1549-1555.

[14] Food and Agricolture Organization of the United Nations (2002). The nutrition transition and obesity. Available at: *http://www.fao.org/ FOCUS/E /obesity /obes2.htm*. Accessed March 8, 2007.

[15] International Obesity Taskforce and European Association for the Study of Obesity (2002). Available at: *http://www.iotf.org/media/euobesity.pdf*. Accessed March 7, 2007.

[16] Must, A., & Anderson, S. E. (2003). Effects of obesity on morbidity in children and adolescents. *Nutrition in Clinical Care, 6(1),* 4–12.

[17] Guo, S. S., Wu, W., Chumlea, W. C., & Roche, A. F. (2002). Predicting overweight and obesity in adulthood from body mass index values in childhood and adolescence. *Am. J. Clin. Nutr, 76,* 653-658.

[18] Whitaker, R. C., Wright, J. A., Pepe, M. S., Seidel, K. D. & Dietz, W. H. (1997). Predicting obesity in young adulthood from children and parental obesity. *New Engl. J. Me, 337*, 869-873.

[19] Must, A., & Strauss, R. S. (1999). Risk and consequences of childhood and adolescent obesity. *Int. J. Obes. Relat. Metab. Disord, 23 (suppl 2),* S2-S11.

[20] Dietz, W. H. (1998). Health consequences of obesity in youth: childhood predictors of adult disease. *Pediatrics,101,* 518-525.

[21] Gordon-Larsen, P., Adair, L. S., Nelson, M. C., & Popkin, B. M. (2004). Five-year obesity incidence in the transition period between adolescence and adulthood: the National Longitudinal Study of adolescent health. *Am. J. Clin. Nutr, 80,* 569-575.

[22] Whitaker, R. C., Wright, J. A., Pepe, MS., Seidel, K. D., & Dietz, W. H. (1997): Predicting obesity in young adulthood from children and parental obesity. *New Engl. J. Med, 337*, 869-873.

[23] Gill, T. P. *(*19979. Key issues in the prevention of obesity. *Br. Med. Bull, 53 (2),* 359-388.

[24] Garn, S. M. *(*1985). Continuities and changes in fatness from infancy through adulthood. *Curr. Prob. Pediatr, 15,* 1-47.

[25] Rolland-Cachera, M. F., Deheeger, M., Bellisle, F., Sempe, M., Guillound-Battaille, M., & Patois, E.. (1984). Adiposity rebound in children: a simple indicator for predicting obesity. *Am. J. Clin. Nutr, 39*, 129-135.

[26] Whitaker, R. C., Pepe, M. S., Wright, J. A., Seidel, K. D., & Dietz, W. H. (1998). Early Adiposity Rebound and the Risk of Adult Obesity. *Pediatrics, 101 (3)*, E5.

[27] Speiser, P. W., Rudolf, M. C., Anhalt, H., Camacho-Hubner, C., Chiarelli, F., Eliakim, A., Freemark, M., Gruters, A., Hershkovitz, E., Iughetti, L., Krude, H., Latzer, Y., Lustig, R. H., Pescovitz, O. H., Pinhas-Hamiel, O., Rogol, A. D., Shalitin, S., Sultan, C., Stein, D., Vardi, P., Werther, G. A., Zadik, Z., Zuckerman-Levin, N., & Hochberg, Z. (2005). Consensus development on childhood obesity. *J. Clin. Endocrinol. Metab, 90(3),* 1971-1887.

[28] Ogden, C. L., Flegal, K. M., Carroll, M. D., & Johnson, C. L. (2002) Prevalence and trends in overweight among US children and adolescents, 1999–2000. *JAMA*, *288,* 1728–1732.

[29] Wang, Y., Monteiro, C., & Popkin, B. M., (2002). Trends of obesity and underweight in older children and adolescents in the United States, Brazil, China, and Russia. *Am. J. Clin. Nutr, 75 (6),* 971-977.

[30] Magarey, A. M., Daniels, L. A., & Boulton, TJC. (2001). Prevalence of overweight and obesity in Australian children and adolescents: reassessment of 1985 and 1995 data against new standard international definitions. *Med. J. Aust, 174*, 561-564.

[31] Ebbeling, C. B., Pawlak, D. B., & Ludwig, D. S. (2002). Childhood obesity: public-health crisis, common sense cure. *Lancet*, *360,* 473-482.

[32] Bellizzi, M. C., Horgan, G. W., Guillame, M., & Dietz, W. H. (2002). Prevalence of childhood and adolescent overweight and obesity in Asian and European countries. In Ed. Nestec Ltd. And Lippincott Williams Et Wilkins. W.H.D Chunming Chen, *Obesity in childhood and adolescence (23-25)*. Philadelphia,.

[33] International Obesity Task Force (2005). EU Platform on Diet, Physical Activity and Health. Available at. *http://ec.europa.eu/health/ph_determinants/life_style/nutrition/documents/iotf_en.pdf.* March, 11 2007.

[34] Lobstein, T., & Frelut, M. L. (2003). Prevalence of overweight among children in Europe. *Obes. Rev, 4,* 195-200.

[35] Marras, V., Macchis, R., Foschini, M. L., Pilia, S., Sortino, M., Tilocca, S., Casini, M. R., Porcu, M., Faedda, A., & Loche, S. (2006). Prevalence of overweight and obesity in primary school children in southern Sardinia, Italy. *Ital. J. Pediatr, 32,* 251-255.

[36] Celi, F., Bini, V., De Giorgi, G., Molinari, D., Faraoni, F., Di Stefanoi, G., Bacosi, M. L., Berioli, M. G, Contessa, G. & Falorni, A. Epidemiology of overweight and obesità among school children and adolescents in three provinces of central Italy, 1993-2001: study of potential influencing variables. *Eur. J. Clin. Nutr, 57,* 1045-1051.

[37] Maffeis, C., Consolaro, A., Cavarzere, P., Chini, L., Banzato, C., Grezzani, A., Silvani, D, Salzano, G., De Luca, F., & Tato, L. (2006). Prevalence of overweight and obesità in 2- to 6-year-old italian children. *Obesità, 14 (5),* 765-769.

[38] Albertini, A., Tripodi, A., Fabbri, A., Mattioli, M. & al (2007). Prevalence, determinants and indicators of risk of obesity in six-year-old children living in Central-North Italy. *Obes. Rev,* (submitted for publication).

[39] Vignolo, M., Pistorio, A., Torrisi, C., Parodi, A., Grassi, S. & Aicardi, G. (2004). Overwiight and obesità in a group of italian children and adolescents:prevalence estimates using different reference standard. *Italian J. Pediatr, 30,* 53-57.

[40] Tripodi A, Daghio MM, Severi S, Ferrari L, and Ciardullo AV. (2005). Surveillance of dietary habits and lifestyles among 5-6 years-old children and their families living in Central-North Italy. *Soz.-Präventivmed, 50,* 134-141.

[41] Cacciari, E., Milani, S., & Balsamo, A., et al (2002). Italian cross-sectional growth charts for height, weight and BMI (6-20 y). *Eur. J. Clin. Nutr, 56,* 171-180.

[42] Reilly, J. J. (2004). Childhood obesità – the global epidemic. *Ital J Pediatr, 30,* 293-298.

[43] Lyon, HN., & Hirschhorn, J. N. (2005). Genetics of common form of obesity: a brief overview. *Am. J. Clin. Nutr, 82 (suppl),* 215S-217S.

[44] American Academy of Pediatrics.(2003) Prevention of pediatric overweight and obesity. *Pediatrics, 112 (2),* 424-430.

[45] Drewnowski, A., & Darmon, N (2005). The economics of obesity: dietary energy density and energy cost. *Am. J. Clin. Nutr, 82 (suppl),* 265S-273S.

[46] Larrañaga, N., Amiano, P., Arrizabalaga, J. J, Bidaurrazaga, J., & Gorostiza, E. (2007). National prevalence of obesity. Prevalence of obesity in 4-18-year-old population in the Basque Country, Spain. *Obes Rev*, doi: 10.1111/j.1467-789X.2006.00306.x

[47] Strauss, R. S., & Knight, J. (1999). Influence of the home environment on the development of obesity in children. *Pediatrics, 103 (6),* 85-92.

[48] Darmon, N., Ferguson, E. L. & Briend, A. (2002). A cost constraint alone has adverse effects on food selection and nutrient density: an analysis of human diets by linear programming. *J. Nutr, 132,* 3764-3671.

[49] Krebs-Smith, S. M., Cook, A., Subar, A. F., Cleveland, L., Friday, J., & Kahle, L. L. (1996). Fruit and vegetable intakes of children and adolescents in the United States. *Arc. Pediatr. Adolesc. Med, 150,* 81-86.

[50] Neumark-Sztainer, D., Story, M., Resnick, M. D. & Blum, R. W. (1996) Correlates of inadequate fruit and vegetable consumption among adolescents. *Prev. Med, 25,* 497-505.

[51] Darmon, N., Ferguson, E. L. & Briend, A. (2003). Do economic constraints encourage the selection of energy dense diets? *Appetite, 41,* 315-322.

[52] Rose, D., & Oliveira, V. (1997). Nutrient intakes of individuals from food- insufficient house-holds in the United States. *Am. J. Public Health, 87,* 1956-1961.

[53] World Health Organization (2004). Global strategy on diet, physical activity and health. Fifty-seventh world health assembly.

[54] Jakicic, J. M. & Otto, A. D. (2005). Physical activity considerations for the treatment and prevention of obesity. *Am. J. Clin. Nutr, 82 (suppl),* 226S-229S.

[55] Prentice, A. M. & Jebb, S. A. (1995). Obesity in Britain: gluttony or sloth? *BMJ, 311,* 437-439.

[56] Dunn, A., Marcus, B., Kampert, J., Garcia, M., Kohl, H. III, & Blair, S. (1999). Comparison of lifestyle and structured intervention to increase physical activity and cardiorespiratory fitness. *JAMA, 281,* 327-334.

[57] Epstein, L. H., Saelens, B. E., Myers, M. D. & Vito, D. (1997). Effects of decreasing sedentary behaviors on activity choice in obese children. *Health Psycol, 16,* 107-113.

[58] Yamanouchi, K., Takashi, T., Chikada, K., & A. L. (1995). Daily walking combined with diet therapy is a useful means for obese NIDDM patients not olnly to reduce body weight but also to improve insulin sensitivity. *Diabetes Care, 18,* 775-778.

[59] Strong, W. B., Malina, R. M., Blimkie, C. J., Daniels, S. R., Dishman, R. K., Gutin, B., Hergenroeder, A. C., Must, A., Nixon, P. A., Pivarnik, J. M., Rowland, T., Trost, S. G., and Trudeau, F. (2005). Evidence based physical activity for school-age youth. *Journal of Pediatrics, 146,* 732-737.

[60] Berkey, C. S., Rockett, HRH., Field, A. E., Gillman, M. W., Lindsay Frazier, A., Camargo, Jr C. A., & Colditz, G. A. (2000). Activity, dietary intake, and weight changes in a longitudinal study of preadolescent and adolescent boys and girls. *Pediatrics, 105,* 56-64.

[61] Andersen, R. E., Crespo, C. J., Bartlett, S. J., Cheskin, L. J., & Pratt, M. (1998). Relationship of physical activity and television watchinh with body weight and level of fatness among children. *JAMA, 279,* 938-942.

[62] Taveras, E. M., Berkey, C. S., Rifas-Shiman, S. L., Frazier, A. L., Colditz, G. A., & Gillman, M. W. (2007). Longitudinal relationship between television viewing and leisure-time physical activity during adolescence. *Pediatrics, 119 (2),* e314-e319.

[63] Matheson, D. M., Killen, J. D., Wang, Y., Varady, A., & Robinson, T. N. (2004). Children's food consumption during television viewing. *Am. J. Clin. Nutr, 79,* 1088-1094.

[64] Borzekowski, D. L., & Robinson, T. N. (2001). The 30-second effect: an experiments revealing the impact of television commercials on food preferences of preschoolers. *J. Am. Diet. Assoc, 101,* 42-46.

[65] Jeffery, R. W, & French, S. A. (1998). Epidemic obesity in the United States: are fast foods and television viewing contributing? *Am. J. Public Heath, 88,* 277-280.

[66] Temple, J. L., Giacomelli, A. M., Kent, K. M., Roemmich, J. N., & Epstein, L. H. (2007). Television watching increases motivated responding for food and energy intake in children. *Am. J. Clin. Nutr;* 85, 355-361.

[67] Doak, C. M., Visscher, TLS., Renders, C. M., & Seidell, J. C. (2006). The prevention of overweight and obesity in children and adolescents: a rewiew of interventions and programmes. *Obes. Rew, 7,* 111-136.

[68] Sharma, M. (2006). School-based intervention for childhood and adolescent obesity. *Obes. Rew, 7,* 261-269.

[69] Summerbell, C. D, Waters, E., Edmunds, L. D., Kelly, S., Brown, T., & Campbell, K. J. (2006). Intervention for preventing obesity in children. *The Cochrane Database of Systematic Rewiews,* Issue 4.

[70] Flynn, M., Mc Neil, D., Tough, S., Maloff, B., Ford, C., Mutasingwa, D. & Wu, M. (2006). Reducing obesity and related chronic disease risk in children and youth: a syntesis of evidence with "best practice" recommendations. *Obes. Rew, 7 (suppl 1),* 7-66.

[71] Robinson, T. N. (1999). Reducing children's television viewing to prevent obesity. *JAMA, 282,* 1561-1567.

[72] Lister-Sharp, D., Chapman, S., Stewart-Brown, S. & Sowden, A. (1999). Health promoting schools and health promotion in schools: two systematic reviews. *Health Tecnol. Assess*, 3 *(22).*

[73] Blanchette, L., & Brug, J., (2005). Determinants of fruit and vegetable consumption among 6-12-year-old children and effective interventions to increase consumption. *J. Hum. Nutr. Dietet, 18,* 431-443.

[74] Perry, C. L., Bishop, D. B., Taylor, G., Murray, D. M., Warren Mays, R., Dudovitz, B.S., Smyth, M. & Story, M. (1998). Changing fruit and vegetable consumption among children: the 5-a-day power plus program in St. Paul, Minnesota. *Am. J. Public Health, 88 (4),* 603-609.

[75] Toschke, A. M., Küchenhoff, H., Koletzko, B., & Von Kries, R. (2005). Meal frequency and childhood obesity. *Obesity Research, 13 (11),* 1932-1938.

[76] Bandura, A. (1986). *Social foundation of thought and action*. Prentice Hall: Englewood Cliffs, NJ.

[77] Müller, M. J., & Danielzik, S. (2007). Childhood overweight: is there need for a new societal approach to the obesity epidemic? *Obes. Rev, 8,* 87-90.

[78] Swinburn, B. & Egger, G. (2002). Preventive strategies against weight gain and obesity. *Obes. rev, 3,* 289-301.

[79] WHO Europe (2006). Gaining health. The European strategy for the prevention and control of noncommunicable diseases. Available at: *http://www.euro.who.int/ Document/ RC56/edoc08.pdf.* Accessed April 10, 2007.

[80] Ferro-Luzzi, A. & Leclercq, C. (1993). Nutritional surveillance: an outline. In: Food and Nutrition Policy in Europe, eds. Van der heij DG, Lowik MRH, Ochuisen T. The Hague Wageningen: *Pudoc Scientific,* 113-117.

[81] Willet, W. C., Sacks, F., Trichopoulou, A., Drescher, G., Ferro-Luzzi, A., Helsing, E., and al. (1995). Mediterranean diet pyramid: a cultural model for healthy eating. *Am. J. Clin. Nutr, 61 (suppl 6),* S1 402-406.

[82] Trichopoulou, A., Orfanos, P., Norat, T., Bueno-de-Mesquita, B., Ocké, M., Peeters, P. H., & al (2005). Modified Mediterranean diet and survival: EPIC-ederly prospective cohort study. *BMJ,* doi:10.1136/bmj.38415.644155.8f.

[83] Frank, B., Hu (2003). Plant based foods and prevention of cardiovascolar disease: an overview. *Am. J. Clin. Nutr, 78,* 544S-551S.

[84] Riboli, E. & Norat, T. (2003). Epidemiologic evidence of the protective effect of fruit and vegetable for cancer risk. *Am. J. Clin. Nutr*; *78,* 559S-569S.

[85] Prior, R. L. (2003). Fruits and vegetables in the prevention of cellular oxidative damage. *Am. J. Clin. Nutr, 78,* 570S-578S.

[86] Feng, J. H., Caryl A. N., & Graham, A. McG (2006). Fruit and vegetable consumption and stroke: meta-analysis of cohort studies. *Lancet, 367,* 320-326.

[87] Wang, L. Y., Yang, Q., Lowry, R., & Wechsler, H. (3003). Economic analysis of a school-based obesity prevention program. *Obes. Res, 11 (11),* 1313-1324.

INDEX

A

B

C

D

E

F

G

H

I

L

M

N

W